# Common Blood Tests

## Fourth Edition

# Common Blood Tests

## What Every Patient Must Know About Lab Tests

### 4th Edition

Edited by N.L. Gifford, PhD

TBL, Inc.
Lake Grove, New York
1999

# COMMON BLOOD TESTS

Copyright 1992, 1995, 1996, 1999 by Technical Books for the Layperson, Inc.

4th Edition, 1999

Formerly titled: *Common Blood Tests: Getting Acquainted With Your Lab Results* (1st, 2nd editions)

Cover: UMIC, SUNY at Stony Brook, New York.

The photograph on the front cover is a magnified photograph of blood which has been stained to highlight the details. The cells containing the dark granules are the largest of the white blood cells (granulocytes, probably neutrophils and basophils). Red blood corpuscles surround them, with varying shapes. At this level of magnification, the remaining components of blood (other white blood cells, platelets, proteins, etc.) are too small to be seen.

Printed in the USA by Morris Publishing, Kearney, Nebraska.

**Library of Congress Cataloging-in-Publication Data**

Common blood tests : what every patient must know about lab tests / edited by N.L. Gifford.
– 4th ed.

    p.   cm.

  Includes bibliographical references and index.

  ISBN 1-881818-09-8 (pbk.)

  1.   Blood—Analysis Popular works.  I. Gifford, N. L. (Nancy L.) , 1946-

RB45.C65  1999

616.07'561—dc21                             99-22724

                                                          CIP

# CAN'T FIND A CERTAIN BLOOD TEST?

Let our Research Department help – free of charge!

For any blood test you wish to know about (and cannot find in *Common Blood Tests*), our researchers will track it down for you. We ask only that you make your request in writing and provide a copy of the lab sheet showing the name of the lab and the name of the test. If you have gotten the name from another source, please send a copy of the article or reference. We will respond directly to you and either return or destroy information of a private nature; your inquiry does **not** go into an electronic data base or any other public storage; the *only* person who actually sees private information is the researcher who handles your request. Be sure to include your name, address and telephone number (if we have questions for you).

Send your request to:

Research Department
TBL, Inc.
P. O. Box 391
Lake Grove, NY 11755-0391

Also, if there is an explanation in *Common Blood Tests* that you do not understand, please let us know.

## Acknowledgements
### Fourth Edition

I would like to thank the readers of *Common Blood Tests* for their questions and for their comments about the earlier editions.

I am most grateful to the professional community: those individuals who privately supported the project and the publishers who bring the information to us all (Springhouse Corporation and the Public Citizen Health Research Group are two particularly good examples).

I am equally indebted to a talented editorial, research and production team who made the Fourth Edition possible: Tim Ernandes, Elizabeth Holt, Janet Mount, Georzetta Ratcliffe, Hella Reeves, Frank Smith, and Roberta Taub.

NLG

# CONTENTS

# HOW TO USE THIS BOOK

The most important thing to know is that the laboratory tests are listed alphabetically, starting with **acid phos**phatase and ending with **zinc**.

A boldface name identifies a blood test that appears in *Common Blood Tests* and how it is listed. So, for example, the test for "acid phosphatase" is alphabetically listed as **acid phos**. We have tried to use the most common abbreviations found on lab sheets.

Because one test may have several names, we list all we have found alphabetically throughout the text, and then tell you the name used in *Common Blood Tests* and where to find the test. (If your lab uses yet a different name, TBL would appreciate hearing about it.)

Below is a sample test, using the format you will see throughout the book. Some categories will interest you, others won't. Just use what is helpful to you.

sample test<br>
(full name of test)

**OTHER NAMES**: We have tried to include all the names used by different labs or medical reference books.

**DESCRIPTION**: Type of substance and its function. This category briefly explains what's being tested in terms that will let you imagine where it is in your body and what it's doing.

**TEST TYPE**: All of the tests in this volume are *blood function* tests. This category tells where the blood is taken from:
- *venous* blood is drawn from the vein

- *capillary* or *peripheral* blood is a drop taken from a fingertip, earlobe or heel (of an infant)
- *arterial* blood is drawn from an artery (usually at the wrist)

Most of the tests also belong to a specific *type* of blood test listed below. They are included here because your lab sheet may mention them.

- **chemistry**
- **hematology**
- **rheology**
- **serology**

**TEST OF**: This indicates which organ or process is involved:

| | |
|---|---|
| endocrine glands | liver |
| heart | metabolism |
| kidney | respiration |

**TEST FOR**: A blood level (of a substance), the appearance (of a cell), or the presence (of an antibody). In other words, when you read the NORMAL values, you can quickly re-check this category to remind yourself what those values refer to.

**HOW OFTEN**: "Regular physical exam" or "screening" refers to tests ordered to assess general health: there may be no symptoms or complaints. Your own health history should determine when you need a physical; otherwise:

to age 30, every 3-5 years
ages 30-50, every 2 years
over age 50, every year

"With symptoms" means that the doctor either suspects a particular problem or wants to rule it out. Your symptoms will guide his/her choice.

**NORMAL**: Includes the widest possible range of values from the laboratories polled. Therefore, our 'normal' range will usually be larger than that of your lab. Always use the range given by your lab. Note, too, that the units of measurement vary considerably; we have tried to include those most commonly used (the list of abbreviations is on page 4).

**HIGH/LOW**: What disease or problem can give rise to higher (or lower) than normal values. Again, we are not diagnosing nor do we want to alarm you. However, our readers have found it helpful to know the kinds of illness associated with abnormal values.

**FALSE HIGH** (or **LOW**): May result from "outside influences." In other words, your results may be deceptively high (or low) because of medication you were taking or something you were doing (jogging, for example).

We have tried to list as many of these variables as we can, again using our imprecise, everyday language. "Hypertension medication" is avoided when we can say "blood pressure reducer" referring to the drugs prescribed for high blood pressure. These variables are categorized as: diet or nutrition: often excesses or deficiencies will affect test values; drugs: over-the-counter or prescription (usually only the generic name is given); environment: non-drug substances or conditions (breathing polluted air or being pregnant, for example); medical tests: some tests will affect the outcome of another test within a certain amount of time.

**COMMENTS**: *Remember, test results of high or low WITHOUT symptoms are rarely significant.*

## MEASUREMENTS:

l:          liter
dl:         deciliter = 1/10 of a liter = 100 milliliters
ml:         milliliter = 1/1,000 liter
μl, mcl:    microliter = 1/1,000,000 liter = $mm^3$
fl:         femtoliter = $10^{-15}$ liter

g:          gram
mEq:        milliequivalent = g/1 ml
μg, mcg:    microgram = 1/1,000,000 g = 1,000 ng
ng:         nanogram = 1,000 pg
pg:         picogram

mol:        mole = mg/100 ml
mmol, mM:   millimole = 1/1,000 mol

mm:         millimeters
$mm^3$:     cubic millimeters = μl
mmHg:       millimeters of mercury (pressure measure)
μ, Mμ:      micron, micrometer = $10^{-6}$ m

U:          unit
IU:         international unit
μU, mcU:    microunits
Other unit standards (e.g., Bessey-Lowry) are designated as
follows:  U/ml (Bessey-Lowry)

## acid phos
## (acid phosphatase)

OTHER NAMES: prostatic acid phosphatase, male PAP test

DESCRIPTION: The *prostate gland* in men secretes fluids which protect and nourish sperm. The gland itself is wrapped around the bottom of the bladder (where the *urethra* begins, the tube which carries either semen or urine out of the body).

An enzyme is a protein which activates the chemical reactions in the body. **Acid phos**phatase is an enzyme of the prostate. If the prostate enlarges, your doctor will check your level of **acid phos** to help diagnose the cause of the growth.

**Acid phos** is also found, to a lesser extent, in the liver, spleen, red blood cells, bone marrow, and platelets. This is why the test is sometimes used as a **tumor marker** (elevated levels can be caused by tumors associated with prostate cancer, leukemia, bone cancer).

TEST TYPE:     venous blood, chemistry

TEST OF:        prostate gland

TEST FOR:      level in blood

HOW OFTEN:   abnormality of prostate

NORMAL:        0.0 - 0.63 U/l (Bessey-Lowry) or
                      0 - 2 U/l (Bodansky) or
                      0 - 5 U/l (King-Armstrong) or
                      0.5 - 1.9 IU/l. *Consult range given by your lab.*

## 6 COMMON BLOOD TESTS

HIGH:                     anemia, blood clots, bone disease, cancer, diabetes,
                          Gaucher's disease, heart attack, hepatitis, kidney
                          disease, Paget's disease, overactive parathyroid,
                          pneumonia, prostate disorder (tumor** or tissue
                          damage), sickle-cell disease

FALSE HIGH:

- drugs: cholesterol reducers (clofibrate), androgen hormones (in women*)
- environment: stimulation of the prostate (exam, enema, etc.) within 48 hours of blood test

FALSE LOW:

- drugs: alcohol
- environment: fluorides, oxalates

COMMENTS:  *Women may receive this test after rape to determine the presence of semen.

**If a prostate tumor has spread to the bones, you will have high **alk phos** levels as well (page 19).

This is not the same test as the **PSA** (prostate-specific antigen) test, page 163.

## adrenal glands function

See individual tests:

| of electrolytes | of hormones |
|---|---|
| **chloride** | **aldosterone** |
| **potassium** | catecholamines |
| **sodium** | **cortisol** |
| | **estrogen** |

DESCRIPTION: The adrenal glands are part of the endocrine system which produces the powerful hormones governing cell activity of the body. They sit on top of our kidneys (one per kidney).

The outer *adrenal cortex* produces sex hormones (androgen, **estrogens**), the hormone **aldosterone** (which regulates the levels of sodium and water in the body), and metabolic hormones (such as **cortisol**) which increase energy, respond to stress, and help to regulate blood pressure.

The middle portion of the adrenal glands, the *adrenal medulla,* produces and stores catecholamines -- hormones that prepare the body for "fight or flight": increase heart rate, constrict blood vessels, redistribute circulating blood (to muscles, brain, heart, kidneys), activate reserves of energy, heighten alertness.

The reason for checking **chloride, potassium** and **sodium** is that normal levels suggest that your adrenal glands are okay and abnormal values suggest where there might be a problem.

TEST TYPE:      venous blood, chemistry

TEST OF:        adrenal glands

TEST FOR:       level of hormones in blood

HOW OFTEN:    with symptoms of hormone imbalance

COMMENTS: DHEA (dehydroepiandrosterone) is a steroid secreted by the adrenals and converted into hormones that are used nearly everywhere: sex organs, placenta, lungs, skin, brain. Levels decline as we age. Predictably, then, replacement of DHEA is touted as an anti-aging strategy. However, one should question whether stimulation of unknown and dormant genes is wise.

**a/g ratio**
(albumin/globulin ratio)
See **protein**, page 162.

# AFP
## (alpha-fetoprotein)

OTHER NAMES: MSAFP (maternal serum alpha-fetoprotein)

DESCRIPTION: This is a blood protein produced by the liver of a fetus. (It is the embryonic version of **albumin** and **globulin**.)
It is a common test of fetal development, sometimes automatically included in a "triple test," an initial screen for fetal abnormalities which consists of **AFP**, unconjugated **estriol**, and **hCG**.

| | |
|---|---|
| TEST TYPE: | venous blood, chemistry |
| TEST OF: | fetus, liver |
| TEST FOR: | level of protein in blood |
| HOW OFTEN: | during pregnancy, 16 to 18 weeks after last menstrual period |
| NORMAL: | 0 - 10 ng/ml nonpregnant adults<br>up to 250 ng/ml during pregnancy. *Consult range given by your lab.* |
| HIGH: | possible defects in developing fetus, particularly with the spinal cord and brain;<br>in nonpregnant persons: cancer (liver, testes – see COMMENTS on the next page, gastric, kidney, lung) |
| FALSE HIGH: | twins, further along in pregnancy (fetus is older) |

LOW:                possible chromosomal problems in fetus (e.g., Down syndrome)

FALSE LOW:       not as far along in pregnancy as thought (fetus is younger)

COMMENTS: Because of its low rate of accuracy (60%), AFP has come under criticism as unnecessarily alarming parents. However, conclusions about fetal health are not drawn solely from an AFP test: if levels are high, further examination (with *ultrasound* and *amniocentesis*) is needed before diagnosis can be made.

Non-pregnant adults may be tested when liver cell cancer or testicular cancer is suspected. For that reason, it is known as a *tumor marker*. However, AFP would not be used to screen the general population for either cancer.

The male gonad is a gland which sits inside the scrotum; it is known either as a "testis" or a "testicle" (usually referred to in the plural as "testes" or "testicles). Less common is another name, "testiculus" (the plural is "testiculi"). They are the male equivalent of ovaries.

# AIDS
## (acquired immune deficiency syndrome)

DESCRIPTION: The last stage of an illness which starts with a virus (HIV) attacking white blood cells, thereby reducing the ability to fight disease. AIDS can be thought of as the absence of enough white blood cells to stop the progress of disease.

AIDS is a *syndrome* which means a set of conditions which must be present for a diagnosis of AIDS to be made. For adults, the Centers for Disease Control (CDC) in Atlanta suggest the following:

- you test positive for HIV
- your CD4+ T-lymphocyte count falls below 200 mm$^3$ or less than 14% of the total lymphocyte count
- you have one or more AIDS-indicating conditions, including *opportunistic* infections* (from germs normally found in the body or the environment)

TEST TYPES:
- HIV status: **antibody** tests (**ELISA, Western blot**, IFA types) or direct viral detection tests (by culture, PCR, HIV-1 p24)
- lymphocyte level: **WBC diff**(erential)
- AIDS-indicating conditions: **antibody** tests for a specific pathogen

HOW OFTEN: as needed for diagnosis and drug therapy

COMMENTS: *Most of the infections associated with AIDS can be diagnosed with an **antibody** test. The italicized names will help you recognize the test name on the lab sheet or help you request information about specific tests.

Parasites: a type of pneumonia (*Pneumocystic carinii pneumonia*), inflammation of the brain (*Toxoplasma gondii*), diarrhea lasting more than a month (from *Cryptosporidium, Isospora hominis* or *Isospora belli*).

Viruses: a herpes-type virus mostly affecting the eye (*Cytomegalovirus*, CMV, which can also affect other organs), cold sores in the mouth or genital blisters (*Herpes simplex* which may also cause bronchitis, pneumonia or infection of the esophagus), *JC virus* which causes many harmless childhood illnesses but can reactivate to cause "progressive multifocal leukoencephalopathy," and perhaps *AIDS dementia complex* which may be caused by HIV invasion of the brain.

Bacteria: tuberculosis (from *Mycobacterium tuberculosis*), "MAI"-induced attacks on other parts of the body (*Mycobacterium avium-intracellulare*), and *Mycobacterium kansasii* or any other strain causing infection. *Salmonella*, a bacterium causing persistent infection, was added to the list in 1995.

Fungi: sores in the mouth which can also appear in the brain (*Candida albicans*), impaired swallowing (*Candidal esophagitis*), fungal meningitis (*Cryptococcus neoformans*, which may also infect the lungs), lung infections (*Histoplasma capsulatum* and *Coccidioides immitis*, both of which can then move throughout the body).

In all these cases, an **antibody** test may help diagnose the infection. However, there is no blood test for *AIDS dementia complex*; diagnosis in generally made by observing reduced mental function in someone who is HIV positive.

Cancer (*Kaposi's sarcoma*, lymphomas, and cancer of the cervix) also counts as evidence of AIDS. Diagnosing cancer is usually indirect, monitoring blood levels when symptoms are present or looking for "cancer markers" (substances in the blood which are associated with a particular type of malignancy).

"Recurrent pneumonia" (whatever the origin) and "wasting syndrome due to HIV" (persistent ill health for more than a month

**AIDS** (cont.)

including fatigue, weight loss, fever, diarrhea) have been added to the list of AIDS-defining infections.

Testing: Where you live will determine how easy it is to get tested. In New York state, AIDS clinics will draw your blood anonymously and free of charge. They send the sample to the Health Department and get the results. You usually have to return to the clinic in person for the results.

Testing may be mandatory when applying for health insurance, life insurance, employment, or when donating blood. The legality of this is being debated.

Remember, sexually active males should always use *latex* condoms with a water-based spermicide during sex.

Further information about the blood tests for and diagnosis of AIDS can be found in TBL's pamphlet *Testing for HIV: What Your Lab Results Mean*, available from the publisher.

## albumin

**(serum albumin)**

DESCRIPTION:  Primary blood protein produced by the liver. It is in the fluid part of the blood (the *plasma*) and keeps the water content of the plasma over 90%. Albumin maintains how thick or thin the blood is (so affects blood pressure). It also maintains water balance between blood and tissue (so controls the volume of plasma).

Albumin levels are added to **globulin** levels to arrive at a measurement of **total protein**. Too little albumin in the blood can cause low **calcium** levels.

TEST TYPE:     venous blood, chemistry

TEST OF:      liver, kidney

TEST FOR:     level in blood

HOW OFTEN:   regular physical exam

NORMAL:     3.2 - 5.6 gm/dl. *Consult range given by your lab.*

HIGH:        tumors, dehydration

FALSE HIGH:  <u>medical tests</u>: BSP (see page 214) within 48 hours before blood test

LOW:        blood protein disorder, burns, cancer, collagen diseases, diarrhea, Hodgkin's disease, kidney disease, liver disease, lupus, malabsorption, malnutrition, peptic ulcer, rheumatoid arthritis, overactive thyroid, water retention (*edema*)

FALSE LOW:

- <u>diet</u>: protein deficiency
- <u>drugs</u>: anticoagulants
- <u>environment</u>: pregnancy, bed rest, intravenous administration of glucose in water

COMMENTS:  Albumin also carries fat from fat deposits to the tissues. Hence, "free fatty acids" (FFA's) can be measured in plasma to evaluate carbohydrate metabolism. Normal levels are 0.19 - 0.90 mEq/l or 8-20 mg/dl.

# alcohol

## (ethyl, isopropyl, methyl)

OTHER NAMES: blood alcohol, ethyl alcohol, ethanol

DESCRIPTION: Drug which is ingested by an individual, either intentionally (as *ethanol* in alcoholic beverages or *methanol* in bootleg liquor) or unintentionally (as *ethylene glycol* or *methanol* in antifreeze, cleaning fluids, industrial solvents or as *isopropanol* which is rubbing alcohol and is used as a disinfectant, liniment or solvent).

Both isopropanol and methanol are more toxic than ethanol. But methanol is less "intoxicating" (inebriating) because it is partially oxidized to formaldehyde in the body. The values below are for ethanol. (Your lab sheet may refer to these forms as "volatiles.")

Most (about 90%) is broken down by the liver, eventually becoming water and carbon dioxide. The remainder stays in its original form and is excreted in breath, sweat and urine. What ultimately causes liver damage is the fact that chronic alcoholics tolerate much higher levels and metabolize ethanol (to *acetaldehyde*) in half the time. It is the high acetaldehyde levels that probably do the damage.

Alcohol noticeably changes the effects of other drugs. The caution against mixing barbiturates with alcohol is the fact that they are metabolized by the same enzyme system which further increases blood levels (and further decreases central nervous system function). Also, persons who regularly use alcohol -- even small amounts every day -- should NEVER use acetaminophen for pain relief.

TEST TYPE:      venous blood, chemistry

TEST OF:        blood

TEST FOR:       presence in blood

## 16 COMMON BLOOD TESTS

HOW OFTEN:    when proof or measure of intoxication is needed; suspected poisoning

NORMAL:    0.00% - 0.05% or
0 - 50 mg/dl. *Consult range given by your lab.*

HIGH:    consumption within hours of test (this can include inhaling ethanol fumes, for example, in a distillery)
- 0.10% - 0.15% or
50 - 100 mg/dl   *legal intoxication*
- above 0.15% or
above 100 mg/dl   *confirms intoxication*
- 0.30% - 35% or
400 - 500 mg/dl   *possible death*

FALSE HIGH:
- drugs: some hypnotics or sedatives (chloral hydrate, glutethimide)
- environment: use of alcohol to prepare the arm for the needle; storage and handling of sample

COMMENTS: Legal definition of intoxication varies from state to state. Biologically, it takes about 30 minutes for a drink of one ounce to get into your bloodstream (15 minutes on an empty stomach) and about 3 hours to leave. At 3 drinks you might be approaching intoxication; in some cases fewer drinks can produce intoxication. Your size, stomach content, gender and many other variables will affect these estimates.

Alcohol is classed as a toxic substance (potentially fatal) of class 2. See **poisoning**, page 140 for a brief explanation of classes.

## aldolase

DESCRIPTION: An enzyme which appears mostly in muscle tissue, helping to produce energy from sugar. It is also found in the heart muscle, liver and red blood cells. Damage will cause the enzyme to leak into the bloodstream.

TEST TYPE:          venous blood, chemistry

TEST OF:            muscle tissue

TEST FOR:           presence in blood

HOW OFTEN:          with suspected tissue damage

NORMAL:             0 - 12 U/ml  *Consult range given by your lab.*

HIGH:               anemia, blood clot, cancer (liver and prostate), DTs (*delirium tremens*), heart attack, hepatitis, lead poisoning, mononucleosis, muscle disease, pancreas infection, physical injury, pneumonia, stroke, richinosis (parasite)

FALSE HIGH:

- drugs: antibiotics, antidepressants (tricyclics), antiinflammatory medication, antipsychotics, arthritis medication, birth control pills, cardio-vascular drugs (beta blocker, blood pressure reducer, heartbeat regulator), cortisone, diabetes medication, gout medication, hormones, narcotics, sedatives, vitamin D
- environment: blood sample held too long before processing, healing bone fracture, pregnancy

## aldosterone
### (serum aldosterone)

DESCRIPTION:  Hormone produced by the adrenal glands, it helps control the balance of electrolytes (**chloride, potassium** and **sodium**) which means helping to maintain blood volume and pressure. If this test is ordered, you should follow a low-carbohydrate, normal-salt diet for the month before the test.

TEST TYPE:  venous blood, chemistry

TEST OF:  kidney

TEST FOR:  level in blood

HOW OFTEN:  with high blood pressure; symptoms of electrolyte imbalance

NORMAL:  1 - 16 ng/dl or
below 20 ng/dl in plasma. *Consult range given by your lab.*

HIGH:  cancer (adrenal tumor), congestive heart failure, high blood pressure, kidney disease, liver disease

FALSE HIGH:

- <u>diet</u>: licorice
- <u>drugs</u>: blood pressure reducers (particularly diuretics and hydralazine), hormones (progesterone)
- <u>environment</u>: exercise, pregnancy, standing just prior to test, stress, surgery

**aldosterone** (cont.)

LOW:                    adrenal gland disease (e.g., Addison's disease), diabetes, toxemia (of pregnancy)

FALSE LOW:        <u>diet</u>: low-salt diet

## alk phos
### (alkaline phosphatase, ALP)

DESCRIPTION:  The liver recycles your blood, cleaning it and re-using what is usable. ALP is an enzyme which appears mostly in the liver and bone. In adults it is usually present in the blood (with more of liver ALP than bone). But damage to either will cause the enzyme to leak into the bloodstream raising normal levels. Used as a **tumor marker** for some cancers of the liver and bone.

It is important to fast for 8 hours, at least, before the test because any fat taken in will stimulate intestinal secretion.

TEST TYPE:        venous blood, chemistry

TEST OF:            liver, bone

TEST FOR:          level in blood

HOW OFTEN:      with symptoms

NORMAL:
- 87 - 250 IU/l for men and women over age 45
- 76 - 196 IU/l for women under age 45

This is a particularly good example of why we recommend paying attention to the range of values on **your** lab sheet. The above range comes from

*Everything You Need To Know About Medical Tests* (see *Bibliography*). Note the extreme differences with the variety of results reported by other sources (including earlier editions of *Common Blood Tests).*

- 20- 130 IU/l or
  0 - 70 U/l (Lange) or
  4 - 13 U/dl (King-Armstrong) or
  1.4 - 4.5 U/dl (Bodansky) or
  0.8 - 2.3 U/dl (Bessy-Lowry)
- Children will show higher values due to active bone growth. *Consult range given by your lab.*

HIGH:                    alcoholism, bile duct obstruction, bone disease, cancer (especially bone cancer), colitis, congestive heart failure, Hodgkin's disease, hormone deficiency, infection (bacterial), liver disease (e.g., hepatitis), parathryroid overactivity, rickets

FALSE HIGH:

- drugs: antibiotics, antidepressants (tricyclics), antiinflammatory medication, antipsychotics, arthritis medication, birth control pills, cardiovascular drugs (beta blockers, blood pressure reducers, heartbeat regulators), cortisone, diabetes medication, gout medication, hormones, narcotics, sedatives, vitamin D
- environment: blood sample held too long before processing, healing bone fracture, pregnancy, eating prior to test

LOW:                     kidney disease, malnutrition, parathyroid under-activity, scurvy

# ALT
## (alanine aminotransferase)

OTHER NAMES: serum glutamic pyruvic transaminase (SGPT), transaminase SGP

DESCRIPTION: ALT is primarily a liver enzyme, although it can be found in other tissue. As an enzyme, it helps to make the liver function as it should: breaking down and storing nutrients. More specifically, it converts amino acids to help produce energy as does AST (page 31). It is often included in the tests ordered to assess your general health.

TEST TYPE:   venous blood, chemistry

TEST OF:   liver, heart

TEST FOR:   level in blood

HOW OFTEN:   regular physical exam

NORMAL:   5 - 30  IU/l or
6 - 36  U/ml (Karmen). *Consult range given by your lab.*

HIGH:   bile duct blockage, heart failure, infection, liver cell damage, liver disease (e.g., hepatitis), mononucleosis

FALSE HIGH:

- <u>drugs</u>: alcohol, antibiotics, antidepressants (tricyclics), antiinflammatory medication, beta blockers, birth control pills, blood pressure reducers, cortisone, gout medication, narcotics

- environment: intake of lead (from pencils or paint chips, for example)

**aluminum**
See **poisoning**, page 140.

### ammonia
### (plasma ammonia, blood ammonia)

DESCRIPTION: When protein is used in the body by the intestines, one of the by-products is ammonia (a nonprotein nitrogen compound). Usually the liver turns the ammonia into *urea* to be excreted by the kidneys. But if the liver isn't working, the ammonia builds up in the body and gets into the blood.

TEST TYPE:     venous blood, chemistry

TEST OF:     liver

TEST FOR:     level in blood

HOW OFTEN:     with symptoms (including abnormal mental states)

NORMAL:     40 - 80 mcg/dl. *Consult range given by your lab.*

HIGH:     bleeding (in stomach), heart failure, liver disease, red blood cell disease, Reye's syndrome

FALSE HIGH:
- diet: high protein diet
- drugs: some diuretics
- environment: prolonged tube feeding

**ammonia** (cont.)

FALSE LOW:

- <u>diet</u>: low protein diet
- <u>drugs</u>: antibiotics (kanamycin, neomycin), laxatives (lactulose)

COMMENTS: The household ammonia we are more familiar with is a toxic substance which should not be in the body.

## amylase
### (serum amylase)

OTHER NAMES: alpha-amylase, ptyalin (salivary amylase) or amylopsin (pancreatic amylase)-- both are the same substance but are sometimes named according to where in the body they are made. Your doctor can order an *amylase fractionation test* to distinguish them.

DESCRIPTION: The pancreas is part of the *gastrointestinal* (GI) system (sitting, roughly, below your stomach and above your small intestine). It is the GI system that transforms what we eat into food for our cells. Amylase is an enzyme that helps digestion by breaking down carbohydrates (starches). It is made in our salivary glands (to begin the process of digestion) and the pancreas. High values of any enzyme mean that it is leaking from the cells/tissues into the bloodstream (from injury or overproduction).

TEST TYPE:       venous blood, chemistry

TEST OF:         pancreas

TEST FOR:        level in blood

HOW OFTEN:    with symptoms; after surgery

NORMAL:    60 - 250 U/dl (Somogyi) or
56 - 190 IU/l. *Consult range given by your lab.*

HIGH:    bile duct obstruction, cancer (ovarian, lung), gallbladder disease, intestinal obstruction, kidney dysfunction, mumps (because of the swelling of the salivary glands), pancreatic disease, salivary gland obstruction, tubal pregnancy (ruptured), ulcers (perforated)

FALSE HIGH:

- <u>drugs</u>: alcohol, antiinflammatory medication, aspirin, diuretics, narcotics, saliva suppressors (those medications which give you a dry mouth)
- <u>environment</u>: anxiety, contamination of sample with saliva

LOW:    liver disease (cirrhosis, hepatitis), pancreatic damage, Parkinson's disease, poisoning (lead or mercury), toxemia (from pregnancy)

FALSE LOW:

- <u>drugs</u>: those which increase the flow of saliva: glaucoma medication, stimulants
- <u>environment</u>: anything which causes drooling

## anion gap

### (serum anion-cation balance)

See individual tests:

- **bicarbonate**
- **chloride**
- **potassium**
- **sodium**

DESCRIPTION: Our blood is slightly alkaline (7.32 – 7.46). All substances in the blood will fall above or below the number 7: those below are *acids*, those above are *alkalis* or "bases." This is measured in the lab by how the substance registers on an electrical scale: acids have a positive charge and are called *cations*, bases are negative and are called *anions*. (An "ion" is simply a molecule having an electrical field.) Our blood, then, carries a slightly negative charge. So long as it stays slightly alkaline, we will be healthy and our blood can do its job. Having the proper **acid-base balance** means keeping within this range.

Normally the amount of sodium and potassium ("anions") together is just a little more than the total amount of bicarbonate and chloride ("cations"). This normal balance can be disrupted by unmeasured anions in the blood (which can come from sulfates, phosphates, ketone bodies, lactic acid, and proteins). These unmeasured anions will affect the normal "gap." But because they are not specifically identified, this test is primarily used for initial screening of a suspected electrolyte imbalance.

TEST TYPE:     venous blood, chemistry

TEST OF:     acid-base balance

TEST FOR:     level in blood by calculation

HOW OFTEN:     with symptoms of acid-base imbalance; when **pH** is abnormal

NORMAL

- 8 - 16 mEq/l
  using the formula $[Na^+ - (Cl^- + HCO_3^-)]$ or
- 10 - 20 mEq/l
  using the formula $[(Na^+ + K^+) - (Cl^- + HCO_3^-)]$
  *Consult range and formula used that is given by your lab.*

HIGH:     metabolic acidosis which may arise from: diabetes, kidney failure, poisoning (from salicylates, methanol, ethylene glycol, paraldehyde), starvation

FALSE HIGH:

- drugs: alcohol, antibacterial (methicillin), anti-inflammatories (corticosteroids, salicylates), bicarbonates, dimercaperol (poison antidote), diuretics (ethacrynic acid, furosemide, hypertension medication, thiazides) epilepsy/gout medication (acetazolamide), hypnotic/sedative (paraldehyde)
- environment: antifreeze (ethylene glycol), prolonged IV infusion of dextrose, rough handling of sample

LOW:     hypermagnesemia (too much magnesium in the blood), tumors (multiple myeloma)

**anion gap** (cont.)

FALSE LOW:

- <u>drugs</u>: antacids (made with magnesium), anti-inflammatories (corticotropin, cortisone), arthritis/gout medication (oxyphenbutazone, phenylbutazone), boric acid, cholesterol reducer (cholestyramine), diabetes medication (chlorpropamide, vasopressin), diuretics (ammonium chloride, others made with mercury or chlorthiazide), lithium

- <u>environment</u>: ingestion of alkalis or licorice, prolonged IV infusion of sodium chloride, rough handling of sample, absorption of iodine from wounds packed with povidone-iodine

### antibody tests

DESCRIPTION: Antibodies (*immunoglobulins*) are protein substances made by white blood cells to get rid of anything foreign in the blood. The body assumes that foreign matter will cause illness.

Generally, once antibodies are made, the threat of illness disappears. For example, a rubella vaccination will cause antibodies to be made which will protect you from getting German measles (also known as *rubella*). This is not, however, true for **HIV** (see page 95), where the presence of antibodies is not protective.

Can the lab test tell whether a *positive* result is protection or infection? More importantly, can you tell from your lab sheet? The actual antibodies are the same in either case. If your lab sheet only gives a negative or positive result and if you have no clinical symptoms, you probably don't have an active infection. Other antibody tests are *quantitative*: the fewer the antibodies, the less likely you are to be actively infected. As we age, we naturally acquire more antibodies. That is why the results of antibody tests are often in "titers" (see page 174) which makes it easier to distinguish immunity from infection.

Tests to determine compatibility: **blood group** and **Rh type** will be used prior to transfusion or transplant. Your lab sheet may refer to *direct Coombs' test* or *indirect Coombs' test*.

Tests to determine the health of your immune system: **WBC diff** will tell you your level of T-cells and B-cells. **Immunoglobulins** (B-cells) will show whether you have normal protection; abnormal levels can be used to help identify specific problems. Your body will announce pregnancy with the presence of **hCG**. More specialized tests can assess the *complement system*.

Reactions to one's own body: All *autoimmune* diseases are of this type. You can develop antibodies to any part of your own body (the organs, the cells, etc.). **RF (rheumatoid factor)** is such a test.

Tests to find viruses: We are most familiar these days with **HIV** and **AIDS**. The tests used to find viruses are **ELISA** and **Western blot** (among others). Your lab sheet will probably give the name of the virus (or condition caused by the virus) that you were tested for: rubella (measles), hepatitis, mononucleosis (your lab sheet may say "mono spot"), Epstein-Barr, herpes, etc.

Tests to find bacteria and fungi: tests for **Lyme disease**, syphilis (your lab sheet may call this a *VDRL* test, Venereal Disease Research Laboratory test), or tuberculosis, for example.

Some labs combine these tests: **TORCH** is frequently required for newborns. Or, a medical condition such as pneumonia can be caused by a virus, a bacterium or fungus, so when you have symptoms your doctor may have to order all three tests to determine how to treat you.

TEST TYPE:      venous blood, serology

TEST OF:         blood

**antibody tests** (cont.)

TEST FOR:        presence of antibody

HOW OFTEN:     with outbreak of disease or known exposure to infection

NORMAL:         negative (low levels may indicate immunity)

POSITIVE:        exposure to disease being tested for

**antibody screening test,** see **Rh type,** page 171.
**antifreeze,** see **poisoning,** page 141.
**antimony,** see **poisoning,** page 141.
**APTT** (activated partial thromboplastin time), see **PTT,** page 165.
**arsenic,** see **poisoning,** page 141.

## arterial blood gases

**(ABG's, blood gases)**
See individual tests for:
- **bicarbonate**
- **carbon dioxide**
- **oxygen**
- **pH**

DESCRIPTION: When the blood travels throughout the body carrying **oxygen,** it is in an *artery*. It returns in a *vein*. If you look at your arm, you may see faint blue lines. These are veins and are blue because the blood is carrying **carbon dioxide** instead of **oxygen.** If you could see arteries in the same way, they would look bright red.

For this series of tests, the blood sample is taken from an artery instead of a vein. This will tell how well the lungs are exchanging carbon dioxide with oxygen.

TEST TYPE:  arterial blood (the sample may be taken from your forearm, upper arm, or thigh)

TEST OF:  lungs

TEST FOR:  level in blood

HOW OFTEN:  with breathing problems or to monitor respiratory therapy; to evaluate damage to heart, kidney or lungs; suspected drug overdose

**aspirin**
See **poisoning**, page 142.

# AST

## (aspartate aminotransferase)

OTHER NAMES: serum glutamic oxalacetic transaminase (SGOT), transaminase SGO

DESCRIPTION: Enzyme found in the liver, heart, muscle, kidney, pancreas. As an enzyme, it helps to make the organs function as they should by regulating the chemical reactions within the organs. There is little reason for it to be in the blood. Damage to the cells of an organ can cause the enzyme to enter the bloodstream which will help your doctor identify where the problem is (particularly in the early stages of liver disease).

TEST TYPE: venous blood, chemistry

TEST OF: heart, liver

TEST FOR: level in blood

HOW OFTEN: with symptoms

NORMAL:
- 1 - 44 IU/l or
  6 - 40 U/ml (Karmen) in adults. *Consult range given by your lab.*
- Substantially higher levels in newborns. Levels in children will follow those in adults.

HIGH: anemia, blood clot, heart attack, liver damage/ disease, muscle injury

FALSE HIGH:

- drugs: antibiotics, antidepressants (tricyclics), antiinflammatory medication, antipsychotics (chlorpromazine), beta blockers, birth control pills, blood pressure medication, blood thinners, cortisone, gout medication, narcotics
- environment: exercise, intake of lead
- medical: injection (shot) into a muscle

**asthma medication**
See **poisoning,** page 142.

**B-cell count**
See B-lymphocytes, page 207 in **WBC diff.**

**bands** (a type of white blood cell)
See page 204 in **WBC diff.**

**barbiturates**
See **poisoning**, page 143.

**barium**
See **poisoning**, page 143.

**basophils**, (a type of white blood cell)
See page 205 in **WBC diff.**

## bicarbonate

### (sodium bicarbonate, HCO₃⁻)

DESCRIPTION: A negatively charged electrolyte, bicarbonate's primary purpose is to regulate the acidity of the blood (see the **pH** test, page 131, as well as the explanation of electrical charge in the **anion gap** test, page 25). It is one of the dissolved components of **carbon dioxide**. In the lungs, the bicarbonate ions return to a gaseous form (carbon dioxide) to be exhaled. Whatever bicarbonate is left in the blood is then excreted through the kidneys.

TEST TYPE:      arterial or venous blood, chemistry

TEST OF:        kidney, lung, metabolism

TEST FOR:       level in blood

HOW OFTEN:      with symptoms

NORMAL:         22 - 25 mEq/l for arterial blood
                21 - 38 mEq/l for venous blood
                *Consult ranges given by your lab.*

HIGH/LOW:       See results in **carbon dioxide**, page 43.

COMMENTS: This is nearly the same test as for *carbon dioxide content* since 90% of the (dissolved) carbon dioxide in the blood is bicarbonate (according to Sobel, page 56, see *Bibliography*). In other words, "normal" for bicarbonate should be about 90% the normal value for carbon dioxide content.

## bilirubin

### (direct, indirect, total)

OTHER NAMES: direct/indirect VandenBergh reaction, bilirubin partition, conjugated/unconjugated bilirubin

DESCRIPTION: *Bilirubin* is a bile pigment (a coloring agent, clear yellow or orange) which is a by-product of the breakdown of **hemoglobin**; bilirubin is carried in the blood to the liver.

On its way to the liver, bilirubin is bound to **albumin** (a protein) in the blood and its measurement is referred to as *indirect* (or unconjugated) *bilirubin*. Further breakdown by the liver "frees" ("conjugates") the pigment which is now referred to as *direct bilirubin*. It is excreted with bile.

The **total** level of bilirubin in the blood is the sum of **direct** and **indirect**. A 4-hour fast should precede the test.

| | |
|---|---|
| TEST TYPE: | venous blood, capillary blood (from infant's heel), chemistry |
| TEST OF: | liver |
| TEST FOR: | level in blood |
| HOW OFTEN: | with symptoms |

**bilirubin** (cont.)

NORMAL:

*Direct*
0.1 - 0.4 mg/d
*Indirect*
0.1 - 0.8 mg/dl
*Total*
- 0.2 - 1.5 mg/dl in adults
- 0.2 - 0.8 mg/dl in children
- 1 - 12 mg/dl in newborns.

HIGH:

Given the proportion of direct to indirect bilirubin, increase of **direct bilirubin** alone will point to some obstruction (e.g., gallstones) in the path from the liver, bile ducts, or gallbladder to the intestines; if the level of **indirect bilirubin** alone is increased, the cause is most likely to be the breakdown of red blood cells from: anemia, enzyme deficiencies, Rh factor incompatibility. If your lab sheet only gives you a **total**: anemia, bile duct obstruction, blood disorder, liver disorder

FALSE HIGH:

- drugs: antibiotics, antiinflammatories, antipsychotics, arthritis medication, blood coagulant, chemotherapy drugs, de-worming drugs, diabetes medication, hormones (male), malaria medication, sedatives, tranquilizers, vitamins A and K, drugs that will make serum orange or yellow
- environment: carotene foods (e.g., carrots), dieting or fasting, methanol (methyl alcohol: antifreeze, solvent, fuel)

## blood

OTHER NAMES: plasma, serum

DESCRIPTION: Blood is the fluid that circulates throughout the body. It carries food, oxygen and other necessary substances to all the organs and tissues in the body. It picks up the garbage (whatever isn't needed) and carries it to disposal sites. Blood also regulates and maintains body temperature, acid-base balance, fluid volume, and protects against infection or poisoning.

Blood tests look at a sample of blood to see what is being carried and how much of it is in the blood. *Normal values* means that what you are looking for is there and is in the amounts that will keep you healthy. When the "values" drop below normal or are much higher than expected, this may be a sign that there is something wrong.

Because the blood goes everywhere in the body (and comes back from everywhere), it can often be used to find out where a problem may exist (which organ, for example, isn't using the nutrition brought by the blood).

COMMENTS: The fluid we call *blood* is actually cells suspended in *plasma.* Roughly, about 64% of the blood we see is plasma, 45% is red blood cells, and less than 1% is white blood cells and platelets. There are about 5½ pints in a 100-pound person, almost 11 pints in a 200-pound person. When the blood clots, the fluid that is left is called *serum* -- plasma without any clotting factors. It is not terribly important to remember these differences for us to understand our blood tests. But sometimes the doctor or lab technician will use the terms.

**blood clotting**
See **platelet aggregation test**, page 138.

## blood group

OTHER NAMES: blood typing, ABO blood type; see also **Rh type**, page 171.

DESCRIPTION; Blood is primarily grouped (identified) according to what proteins are on the surface of the red blood cell. The four most common groups -- those used to determine compatibility -- are **type A, type B, type AB** and **type O** (which has none of the surface identifiers so can be accepted by all other blood types). Once the blood is typed, further compatibility can be determined: whether Rh-positive antibodies are present (*direct* and *indirect Coombs'* tests), whether you have antibodies to white blood cells (*leukoagglutinins* which are detected with a *white cell antibodies test*).

*Crossmatching* is a type of **antibody** detection test used prior to transfusion: the donor's red blood cells are tested with the recipient's serum. The two are compatible if the serum does not destroy the donor's RBC's (i.e., the test is negative). Some lab reports may distinguish *major crossmatching* (compatibility of the donor's red blood cells with the recipient's serum) from *minor crossmatching* (compatibility of the recipient's red blood cells with the donor's serum).

TEST TYPE:   capillary or venous blood, serology

TEST FOR:    blood type

HOW OFTEN:   prior to blood transfusion, during pregnancy

## blood smear

DESCRIPTION: A drop of blood is smeared (from thick to thin) on a slide for examination.

TEST TYPE:     capillary blood, hematology, CBC

TEST FOR:     appearance, cell integrity, frequency of cell types

HOW OFTEN:     regular physical exam

NORMAL:

- platelets: about ½ the size of red blood cells (RBC). See *platelet estimate* (page 139).
- RBC: round without a nucleus, paler center
- WBC: See results of **WBC differential** test (page 202).

ABNORMAL:

- platelets: increase in size or are nearly absent from smear
- RBC: variations in shape, size, color
- WBC: variations within type, abnormal percentages

**blood sugar**
See **glucose** test, page 81.

**bromide**
See **poisoning**, page 143.

# BUN
## (blood urea nitrogen)

OTHER NAMES: urea n; some labs will do a "nonprotein nitrogen" (NPN) test instead of a BUN

DESCRIPTION: The kidneys are part of the recycling system, filtering out fluid waste and returning usable nutrients to the body. *Urea* is the end product of protein breakdown and appears in the blood as *urea nitrogen.* This test measures the portion of nitrogen in urea. This is one of the most common tests performed because it is a quick and inexpensive way to see if your kidneys are working properly.

TEST TYPE:      venous blood, chemistry

TEST OF:        kidney

TEST FOR:       level in blood

HOW OFTEN:      regular physical exam or once every 10 years (more often for males between the ages of 61-70)

NORMAL          5 - 25 mg/dl. *Consult range given by your lab.*

HIGH:           bleeding (GI), dehydration, heart failure, kidney disease, starvation, urinary tract obstruction

FALSE HIGH:

- drugs: antibiotics, antifungal medications, anti-inflammatory medications, asthma medications, blood pressure drugs, diabetes medication, diuretics, sedatives

- environment: exposure to antimony compounds (see page 141), arsenic, burns
- medical: whole blood

LOW: liver disease, malnutrition

FALSE LOW:

- drugs: antibiotic (chloramphenicol)
- environment: excessive fluid intake
- nutrition: protein deficiency

## BUN:creat ratio
### (blood urea nitrogen/creatinine ratio)

TEST TYPE: venous blood, chemistry

TEST OF: kidney

TEST FOR: level in blood

HOW OFTEN: regular physical exam or once every 10 years (more often for males between ages 61-70)

NORMAL 20:1 which means that the BUN level should be 20 times the creatinine level. *Consult range given by your lab.*

HIGH/LOW: See individual tests for **BUN** and **creatinine**.

**cadmium**, see **poisoning**, page 143.
**caffeine**, see **poisoning**, page 144.

## calcium
### (ionized calcium, $Ca^{++}$)

DESCRIPTION: Calcium is the dominant mineral found in our bodies and is stored in our bones. Only 1% - 2% actually circulates in the blood. When the blood levels falls below normal, calcium moves out of the bones and teeth and dissolves in the blood to restore the blood level.

When dissolved in the blood, calcium is "ionized," has an electric charge, which is why it is known as an *electrolyte*. It is measured with serum calcium. See COMMENTS on the next page.

We normally excrete some calcium daily, which is why our diet must include daily servings of calcium-rich foods. But most dietary forms don't dissolve well enough to be taken up by the intestines. The sun and our parathyroid gland together make the substances that will eventually dissolve the calcium so we can use it.

TEST TYPE:    venous blood, chemistry

TEST OF:    kidney, parathyroid gland, metabolism

TEST FOR:    level in blood (total of ionized and non-ionized)

HOW OFTEN:    regular physical exam; with symptoms (nausea, vomiting, dehydration; or numbness, muscle spasms, seizures, irregular heartbeat)

NORMAL:

- 8.8 - 11.5 mg/dl for adults, with higher levels during rapid bone growth
  (4.6 - 5.3 mg/dl ionized)
- 7.4 - 14.0 mg/dl for newborns
  *Consult range given by your lab.*

HIGH:               bone cancer, bone marrow tumor, multiple bone fractures, kidney disease, parathyroid over-activity, respiratory disease, thyroid disorders; see also page 144

FALSE HIGH:

- drugs: antacids
- environment: prolonged bed rest

LOW:               albumin deficiency, bone disorders, Cushing's syndrome, digestive disorders, kidney disease, pancreas disease, parathyroid underactivity

FALSE LOW:

- environment: pregnancy
- medical tests: BSP test (page 214) within 48 hours
- nutrition: too few dairy products, too little vitamin D

FALSE RESULTS (HIGH/LOW): drugs: anticoagulants, birth control pills, diuretics, epilepsy medication, glaucoma medication, hormones, insulin

COMMENTS: The ionized form of calcium is the only useful form, but many labs cannot isolate the two for separate measurement. Where measurements are not given for each, the ionized form probably constitutes about 50% of the total calcium level in the blood. It is possible to measure just the amount of ionized calcium using something called "ion selective electrode" methodology; your lab sheet will have a note if such a specialized test was done.

**cantharides**
See **poisoning**, page 145.

## carbon dioxide, (CO₂)

DESCRIPTION: A waste product of metabolism, carbon dioxide starts out in the body's tissues and is picked up by the blood for disposal. However, most of it travels in the blood in the form of hydrogen ions (attached to the carrier hemoglobin, **Hgb**, in the red blood cell) and **bicarbonate** ions (see page 33).

If the pressure of carbon dioxide in red blood cells is excessive, the gas can spill out of the cells and dissolve in the plasma. *Carbon dioxide tension* (also called the *partial pressure of carbon dioxide* or *pCO₂*) measures the gaseous form of carbon dioxide in the blood. *Carbon dioxide content* (or *capnography*) measures the dissolved $CO_2$ in the blood. *Carbon dioxide combining power* measures how much carbon dioxide the blood *could* hold.

TEST TYPE:      arterial and venous blood, chemistry

TEST OF:        kidney, lung, metabolism

TEST FOR:       level in blood

HOW OFTEN:      with symptoms; to evaluate acid-base balance

NORMAL:         *Carbon dioxide tension, pCO₂*
                 35 - 45 mm Hg for arterial blood
                 38 - 59 mm Hg for venous blood
                 *Carbon dioxide content*
                 19 - 25 mM/l for arterial blood
                 22 - 38 mM/l for venous blood
                 *Carbon dioxide combining power*
                 24 - 32 mEq/l for arterial blood
                 38 - 50 mEq/l for venous blood
                 *Consult ranges given by your lab.*

HIGH:                   acid-base disorders, adrenal gland overactivity, asthma, blood too alkaline, breathing difficulty, central nervous system disorder, chest injury, Cushing's syndrome, drug overdose, emphysema, heart disease, intestinal obstruction, lung disease, starvation

FALSE HIGH:

- drugs: anesthesia, antacids, bicarbonate, cortisone, diuretics, hormones, steroids
- environment: alkaline intake (baking soda), exercise (hand, forearm), licorice, blood sample exposed to air, stomach recently pumped, vomiting

LOW:                    alcohol poisoning, ammonium chloride (a diuretic) poisoning, aspirin poisoning, blood too acid, diabetes, diarrhea, fever, hyperventilation (rapid breathing), intestinal drainage, kidney or liver disease, shock

FALSE LOW:

- drugs: antibiotics (particularly methicillin), aspirin, mercury diuretics, emetic (page 215, e.g., dimercaprol), glaucoma drugs
- environment: antifreeze or methyl alcohol ingestion, diarrhea, overheated room (causing rapid breathing)

COMMENTS: Generally, the $CO_2$ test will be ordered when lung function is being evaluated and the test for **bicarbonate** when kidney function is being evaluated. Results of both tests are enhanced when the blood's **pH** is tested as well.

## carbon monoxide, CO
### (carboxyhemoglobin)

DESCRIPTION: A common gas given off during incomplete combustion (from household heaters, cars, gasoline engines, power lawn mowers, charcoal barbecues, cigarettes, for example). Highly toxic because it binds to hemoglobin, replacing the oxygen.

TEST TYPE:     venous blood, chemistry

TEST OF:       respiration

TEST FOR:      level in blood

HOW OFTEN:     with symptoms or exposure

NORMAL:
- 0% - 3% nonsmokers*
- 5% - 15% smokers
- 8% - 15% frequent and sustained exposure to cars

HIGH:          carbon monoxide poisoning (coma is induced as levels approach 50%; some people are far more sensitive and will be poisoned at lower levels)

COMMENTS: *Of course there should be no carbon monoxide in the body; its presence will always impair respiratory function whether or not there are symptoms (see page 145). *Chronic carbon monoxide poisoning* is far more common in our industrial society. We can maintain levels in our bodies just from the gas in the environment. The next time you are scheduled for a blood test, you might want to ask for a **CO** test just to find out what levels you are living with.

## cardiac function tests

See individual tests:

- ◆ cardiac enzyme studies ("heart attack enzymes")
  - • **AST**
  - • **CK**
  - • **LD**
  - • **renin**
- ◆ **lipid panel**

DESCRIPTION: The heart is responsible for the movement of the blood throughout the body. The health of the heart can, to some degree, be assessed by measuring the level of the enzymes and lipids in the blood. If the heart muscle is injured, the enzymes leak out of the muscle into the bloodstream.

TEST TYPE:        venous blood, chemistry

TEST OF:          heart

TEST FOR:         level in blood

HOW OFTEN:        with symptoms or suspected heart attack

COMMENTS: Enzyme studies can be performed "serially" to determine the extent of damage to the heart muscle. This means that the tests will be repeated at regular intervals to monitor increasing enzyme levels.

# CBC
## (complete blood count)

OTHER NAMES: hemogram

See individual tests:
- **blood smear**
- **HCT** (hematocrit)
- **Hgb** (hemoglobin)
- **platelet estimate**
- **platelet count**
- **RBC**
- **RBC indices**
- **RDW***
- **WBC**
- **WBC differential**

DESCRIPTION: Examination and count of the blood cells (red cells, white cells and platelets).

TEST TYPE:       venous blood, hematology

TEST OF:         whole blood

TEST FOR:        appearance/frequency of cell types

HOW OFTEN:       regular physical exam

COMMENTS: *RDW (red cell distribution width) is a specialized test used once you have been diagnosed with anemia. It will confirm that the source of your anemia is iron deficiency.

## chloride, Cl

### (serum chloride)

DESCRIPTION: An **electrolyte** (having an electrical charge when dissolved in the blood), specifically an *anion*, involved in water balance and acid-base balance of body fluids. It is a chloride ion that can move across the red blood cell membrane and provide transport for the exchange of gases in respiration.

Its presence provides the balance for **sodium** (a *cation*), which is interesting given the fact that chloride comes from salt (sodium chloride) in the diet. It is absorbed through the intestines and excreted through the kidneys.

TEST TYPE: venous blood, chemistry

TEST OF: kidney, adrenal glands

TEST FOR: level in blood

HOW OFTEN: with symptoms of acid-base imbalance

NORMAL: 95 - 103 mEq/l. *Consult range given by your lab.*

HIGH: adrenal gland overactivity, aldosterone hormone excess, coma, dehydration, kidney failure, head injury accompanied by rapid breathing, metabolic acidosis, stupor

FALSE HIGH: environment: rapid breathing (from exercise, high altitude)

**chloride** (cont.)

LOW: Addison's disease, adrenal gland underactivity, dehydration (from burns, diarrhea), diabetes, edema, heart failure (congestive), infection, intestinal obstruction, kidney failure (chronic), metabolic alkalosis

FALSE LOW: environment: heat exhaustion, surgery, prolonged vomiting, gastric suctioning

FALSE RESULTS (HIGH/LOW): drugs: antiinflammatory medication, blood pressure medication, diuretics, sedatives (bromides), steroids

COMMENTS: High chloride values, along with a high sodium in the body's sweat, is an indication of *cystic fibrosis*, a very serious respiratory disease.

**chlorinated pesticides**, see **poisoning**, page 145.
**chlorinated phenols**, see **poisoning**, page 146.

## cholesterol
### (serum cholesterol)

DESCRIPTION: Not a fat but a fatty substance (lipid) used in construction of cell membranes (it strengthens blood vessels), bile acids, and hormones. It can only be carried through the blood if it is attached to a protein (as a *lipoprotein*). Hence, the actual substance measured in the blood is the lipoprotein (see **LDL** and **HDL** tests).

Cholesterol is taken from the food we eat and then transformed into usable substances in the liver and other body tissues. Because so much of our food is processed, we actually take in more *saturated* fat than our bodies can use.

TEST TYPE:      venous blood, chemistry, lipid panel

TEST OF:        heart

TEST FOR:       level in blood

HOW OFTEN:      every 5 years

NORMAL:

- 120 - 280 mg/dl in adults.    (Also,    see **cholesterol:HDL ratio** on the next page.)
- 50 - 100 mg/dl in newborns
- 70 - 175 mg/dl in infants to one year old
- 135 - 240 mg/dl in children. *Consult ranges given by your lab.*

HIGH:           bile obstruction, diabetes, low HDL levels, heart disease, lipid disorders, liver disease, pancreas inflammation, thyroid underactivity

FALSE HIGH:

- <u>diet</u>: eating eggs/brains in the 12-hour period before the test
- <u>drugs</u>: asthma medication, birth control pills, cortisone, diuretics (thiazides), epilepsy medication, male hormones, sedatives, vitamins A & D
- <u>environment</u>: absence of oxygen (high altitudes), pregnancy, rough handling of sample

**cholesterol** (cont.)

LOW:            anemia, infection, liver damage, malnutrition (from starvation), thyroid overactivity

FALSE LOW:

- <u>drugs</u>: antibiotics, aspirin, female hormones, vitamin B$_3$
- <u>environment</u>: fasting

COMMENTS: Movement just prior to the exam may affect values; try to sit during the preceding 5 minutes.

Although levels about 200 may be "normal," they are not considered healthy due to increased risk of heart disease. Similarly, levels below 160 are coming under suspicion as perhaps increasing the risk of colon cancer and stroke. (*New England Journal of Medicine*, vol. 6, April 1989: a study of men with cholesterol levels within the range of 160-220 had substantially fewer deaths from all causes than men with higher and lower cholesterol levels.)

## cholesterol:HDL ratio

DESCRIPTION: This ratio may be a better indicator of heart health than just your cholesterol level. However, you may have to request that the lab measure the level of **HDL** (page 89) as well as cholesterol.

TEST TYPE:      venous blood; arithmetic value from cholesterol and HDL levels (divide your **cholesterol** level by the **HDL** level, <u>cholesterol</u>)
                                    HDL

TEST OF:        heart

TEST FOR:    risk of coronary heart disease

HOW OFTEN:   every 5 years without risk

NORMAL:
- 3.4 for men
- 3.3 for women. *Consult range given by your lab.*

COMMENTS:   Ratios under 4.5 are thought to be quite good. (*Prevention* magazine, March 1989)


## chemistry
### (blood chemistry)

See individual tests:
> *To monitor general health:*
> - **albumin**
> - **ALT**
> - **BUN**
> - **calcium**
> - **cholesterol**
> - **creatinine**
> - **electrolytes**
> - **GGTP**
> - **glucose**
> - **iron studies**
> - **kidney function**
> - **lipase**
> - **uric acid**

**chemistry** (cont.)

*To look for or monitor special problems. For example,*

- **acid phosphatase** (prostate gland)
- **AFP** (fetal health)
- **aldolase** (muscle injury)
- **alk phos** (liver, bone)
- **amylase** (pancreas)
- **bicarbonate** (respiration)
- **CK** (heart)

*To test for drugs, nutrients, toxins, such as*

- **alcohol**
- **carbon monoxide**
- **folic acid**
- **lead**
- **poisoning**

DESCRIPTION: Substances in the blood which can be measured (a "quantitative" test) include: by-products of metabolism, nutrients, fats, enzymes, hormones, proteins, salts, and minerals as well as substances ingested by the individual.

Any **direct** measurement of a substance in the blood is a *chemistry* test (as distinguished from a *serology* test which measures a substance **indirectly** through the presence of antibodies or antigens or a *hematology* test which is a "qualitative" test that looks at the appearance of the blood cells). Drugs, vitamins, toxins, almost anything that gets into the bloodstream, can be measured. Usually *Common Blood Tests* won't list each and every possible substance that can be measured. Your common sense will tell you that if you don't ingest a substance, it won't be in your blood; if you do, it will.

As a general rule, whenever "chemistry" is noted on the TEST TYPE, it is a good idea to fast prior to the test -- even if you are not so instructed. As tests become more and more sensitive, values will be more easily affected by what you ingest in the 10-12 hour period prior to the test.

TEST TYPE:     venous and capillary blood, chemistry

TEST OF:       general health

TEST FOR:      level in blood of specified substances

COMMENTS: A 24-hour urine test is usually included with blood chemistry screening.

# CK

**(serum creatine kinase)**

OTHER NAMES: creatine phosphokinase (CPK)

DESCRIPTION: CK is an enzyme (page 66) which plays a role in the metabolism of *muscle* cells. The values in the NORMAL range reflect the normal wear and tear on muscle tissue. Increased muscle development (from "pumping iron") will result in correspondingly higher values. Infants as well have significantly higher levels.

Since the heart is perhaps our most important muscle, CK can tell us a lot about our heart. It is the first enzyme to increase following a heart attack.

Of course, CK is also in the liver, arm or leg muscle and the brain. Since each of these enzymes differ slightly (CK from the brain is slightly different from CK from the liver), isolating each CK *isoenzyme* can help discover which muscle is damaged. The isoenzymes can be further analyzed for more precise diagnosis by the measurement of subunits called *isoforms*.

TEST TYPE:     venous blood, chemistry

TEST OF:      heart, muscle tissue

TEST FOR:     level in blood

HOW OFTEN:   with symptoms of heart attack

NORMAL:

- 55 - 170 IU/l in men
- 30 - 35 IU/l in women. *Ranges vary dramatically. Use those given by your lab.*

**CK$_1$ (BB)** isoenzyme from the brain:
0 IU/l or 0% of total **CK**
**CK$_2$ (MB)** isoenzyme from the heart:
0-7 IU/l or 0-6% of total **CK**
**CK-MB$_2$** isoform concentration: less than 1.0
**CK-MB$_2$** to **CK-MB$_1$** ratio: less than 1.5
**CK$_3$ (MM)** isoenzyme from the skeletal muscles:
5-70 IU/l or 94-100% of total **CK**

HIGH:    carbon monoxide poisoning, fever (reaction to anesthesia), heart attack, heart disease, heart muscle inflammation, muscle inflammation or injury, potassium deficiency, seizure (from lung or brain damage)
**CK$_1$ (BB)** brain tissue injury, kidney failure, malignant tumors, severe shock
**CK$_2$ (MB)** heart attack, muscular dystrophy (deterioration of the muscles)
**CK$_3$ (MM)** injury (including surgery, intramuscular injection, excessive agitation), underactive thyroid

FALSE HIGH:    <u>environment</u>: exercise, injection into muscle

## clotting factors

DESCRIPTION: *Clotting factors* are inactive proteins, enzymes, that circulate in the blood, ready to respond in a flash to tissue injury.

**Factor I** = fibrinogen

**Factor II** = prothrombin

**Factor III** = tissue thromboplastin, or tissue factor

**Factor IV** = calcium or calcium ions

**Factor V** = proaccelerin, or accelerator globulin, or AcG, or labile factor

**Factor VII** = proconvertin, or stabile (stable) factor, or autoprothrombin I, or serum pro-thrombin conversion accelerator (SPCA)

**Factor VIII** = antihemophiliac factor (AHF), or hemophilia A factor, or antihemophiliac globulin (AHG)

**Factor IX** = plasma thromboplastin component (PTC), Christmas factor, autoprothrombin II

**Factor X** = the Stuart factor, autoprothrombin II, Stuart-Prower factor

**Factor XI** = plasma thromboplastin antecedent (PTA, immature form for plasma thromboplastin)

**Factor XII** = the Hageman factor

**Factor XIII** = fibrin stabilizing factor (FSF)

There is no Factor VI. At one time, accelerin was thought to be a coagulating factor and was named Factor VI. It is unusual for doctors and laboratories to be so specific with consumers about the nuts and bolts of a process. However, HIV contamination of public blood supplies has led to frequent reference to the specific clotting factors in news articles.

TEST TYPE:     venous blood

TEST FOR:      presence of factor

HOW OFTEN:     when a deficiency is suspected; poor wound healing

NORMAL:      a clotting time of 50% - 150% of normal
Factor XIII: normal = "clot stable"

SLOW:        deficiency of a specific factor
**Factor II**: liver disease, vitamin K deficiency; lethal if absent at birth
**Factor V**: liver disease, disseminated intravascular coagulation, fibrinogenolysis
**Factor VII**: liver disease, vitamin K deficiency
**Factor VIII**: hemophilia A, von Willebrand's disease, factor VIII inhibitor, liver disease, tumors, umbilical bleeding in newborns, recurrent bleeding or bruising, prolonged bleeding, bleeding in a joint cavity, miscarriage (rare)
**Factor IX**: hemophilia B, liver disease, factor IX inhibitor, vitamin K deficiency, warfarin therapy
**Factor X**: liver disease, vitamin K deficiency, scattered intravascular coagulation
**Factor XI**: trauma, surgery; sometimes newborns are briefly deficient
**Factor XII**: deficiency may appear briefly in newborns

COMMENTS: Oral anticoagulants are usually stopped before these tests.

## coagulation panel
### (coagulation screening tests)

See individual tests:

- blood clot retraction*
- **clotting factors**
- **fibrinogen**
- **platelet aggregation test**
- **platelet count**
- **pro time**
- **PTT**
- thrombin time

DESCRIPTION: These tests evaluate all the substances involved in blood clotting.

TEST TYPE:     venous blood

TEST OF:     liver

TEST FOR:     clotting capacity

HOW OFTEN:     before surgery, during drug therapy

COMMENTS:  *The clot retraction test monitors separation of a blood clot from the test tube wall (usually 30-60 minutes). The test, performed on a venous blood sample and used to assess platelet function, is not a common one.

**copper**
See **poisoning**, page 146.

## cortisol

### (plasma cortisol)

OTHER NAMES: hydrocortisone, 17-hydroxycortisone

DESCRIPTION: Hormone produced by the adrenal glands from cholesterol. It helps to break down sugar, protein and fat as well as helping to regulate the water in the body (through the regulation of **sodium** and **potassium**). It also assists the immune system against stress, infection and inflammation.

Two samples are needed. Your lab sheet may say "cortisol A.M." or "cortisol P.M." However, it is more important to adjust the timing to your schedule: the first sample after waking up and before you begin your primary daily activities, the second sample about 8 hours later.

TEST TYPE:     venous blood, chemistry

TEST OF:     adrenal gland, pituitary gland, hypothalamus

TEST FOR:     level in blood; comparison of levels from a second sample drawn 8 hours after the first

HOW OFTEN:     at birth; with symptoms

NORMAL:     first sample (before work)
5 - 30 mcg/dl -- if a "total cortisol" level is indicated, it will be the results of this sample
second sample (after work)
2 - 18 mcg/dl -- about a 50% decrease.
*Consult ranges given by your lab.*

**cortisol** (cont.)

HIGH:                Cushing's disease (oversecretion of the adrenal gland)

LOW:                Addison's disease, fungal infection, pituitary gland malfunction (too much androgen), TB

FALSE RESULTS (HIGH or LOW):
- drugs: anticonvulsants (Dilantin), birth control pills, diuretics (spironolactone), estrogens
- environment: obesity, pregnancy, emotional or physical stress

**CPK**, see **CK** (serum creatine kinase) test, page 55.

## creatinine

### (serum creatinine)

DESCRIPTION: When muscle cells absorb nutrients, they create nitrogen (in the form of *creatinine*) as a by-product. The kidney should extract it from the blood and dispose of it as urine. Normal range in the blood will be proportional to one's muscle mass (higher values in a body builder, for example).

The original substance delivered to the muscle is *creatine*. (See, for example, the **CK** test, page 55.) You will be asked to restrict food/fluid for 8 hours before the test.

TEST TYPE:        venous blood, chemistry

TEST OF:          kidney

TEST FOR:         level in blood

HOW OFTEN:     regular physical exam

NORMAL:

- 0.8 - 1.5 mg/dl in men
- 0.5 - 1.0 mg/dl in women
- 0.4 - 1.2 mg/dl in children. *Consult range given by your lab.*

**creatine** as creatinine

0.1 - 0.6 mg/dl in men

0.2 - 1.0 mg/dl in women

HIGH:               growth disorders, intestinal obstruction, kidney disorder/disease, urinary tract obstruction

FALSE HIGH:

- drugs: antibiotics (cephalosporin), barbiturates, sedatives, vitamin C
- medical tests: BSP (page 214) or PSP (page 219) within 48 hours of the blood test

FALSE LOW:     drugs: blood pressure reducer

COMMENTS: *Creatinine clearance* is a urine test called for when a more precise measure of kidney function is needed.

**crossmatching**, see **blood group**, page 37.
**cyanide**, see **poisoning**, page 147.
**DHEA**, see page 8.
**differential white count**, see **WBC diff**, pages 202-209.
**digitoxin** and **digoxin**, see **poisoning**, page 145.
**direct antiglobulin test** (*direct Coombs'*), see **Rh type**, page 171.
**direct bili**, see **bilirubin** test, page 34.
**drug testing**, see **alcohol, poisoning** tests.

## electrolytes

**(anions [-] and cations [+])**

See individual tests:

- **anion gap**
- **bicarbonate**
- **calcium**
- **carbon dioxide***
- **chloride***
- lactic acid
- **magnesium**
- **potassium***
- **sodium**

**\*electrolyte panel: (Na, K, Cl, CO$_2$)**

DESCRIPTION: When dissolved in the blood, some substances become "ionized," take on an electric charge. They are then known as *electrolytes*. Taking on an electric charge means simply that the substance can hold electricity and conduct electricity. When electrolytes are properly combined -- positive particles with negative -- the fluid will be "electrically neutral" or "balanced." **Acid-base balance** is this combination of electrolytes. See **pH** test (page 131).

Consequently, electrolytes are crucial to the functioning of our body's fluids (about 60% of your total body weight): how water is used, maintaining the proper viscosity (**osmolality**), providing the proper environment for nerves and muscles to communicate.

TEST TYPE:      venous blood, chemistry

TEST OF:      acid-base balance

TEST FOR:      level of electrolytes in blood

HOW OFTEN:      with symptoms; when **pH** is abnormal

# ELISA

## (enzyme-linked immunosorbent assay)

DESCRIPTION: A type of test in which enzymes are used to detect the presence of viral antibodies. It is the initial screening test for HIV antibodies in the blood but of course can screen for any number of viruses (depending on which enzymes are used).

TEST TYPE:      venous blood, serology

TEST OF:        blood

TEST FOR:       presence of antibody in blood

HOW OFTEN:      with symptoms of depressed immune function or other disease indicator; exposure to pathogen

NORMAL:         negative

FALSE NEGATIVE: In the case of HIV, it may be too early to detect antibodies (individuals vary widely -- from 4 weeks to 3 years -- to begin antibody production). The likelihood of a false negative depends on your level of risk: high risk individuals have many more false negatives than low risk individuals (who have almost none).

### ELISA (cont.)

ABNORMAL: <u>positive</u>: antibodies present, exposure to pathogen probable

<u>indeterminate</u>: laboratory cannot tell, test should be repeated in 3 months

FALSE POSITIVE:

- laboratory error (including switched samples)
- similarity of other proteins in the blood to the antibody being sought. This is why the **Western blot** (page 209) is used to confirm a positive result.

### endocrine glands

Consists of:

- **adrenal glands**
- hypothalamus
- **ovaries** (female)*
- **pancreas**
- **parathyroid glands**
- **pituitary gland**
- **testes** (male)*
- **thyroid gland**

*Also known as "gonads" or sex organs.

DESCRIPTION: The function of the endocrine system is to produce hormones that regulate the activities of cells.

TEST TYPE: venous blood, chemistry

TEST OF: hormonal balance

TEST FOR: appropriate levels of hormones

HOW OFTEN:    when precise diagnosis is needed

**eosinophils** (a type of white blood cell), see page 205 in **WBC diff**.
**erythrocyte count**, see **RBC** (red blood cell count)  page 166.
**ESR** (erythrocyte sedimentation rate), see **sed rate**, page 172.

## enzymes

See individual tests:

*Genetic screening*
- **galactose transferase**
- **PKU** (phenylketonuria screening)

*Heart*
- **CK** (creatine kinase)
- **LD** (lactate dehydrogenase)

*Kidney*
- **renin**

*Liver*
- **alk phos** (alkaline phosphatase)
- **ALT** (alanine aminotransferase)
- **AST** (aspartate aminotransferase)
- **GGT** (gamma glutamyl transferase)
- **GGTP** (gamma glutamyl transpeptidase)

*Pancreas*
- **aldolase**
- **amylase**
- **lipase**

*Prostate gland*
- **acid phosphatase**
- **PSA** (prostate-specific antigen)

**enzymes** (cont.)

DESCRIPTION: *Enzymes* are an enormous group of highly specialized proteins that regulate the innumerable chemical reactions involved in metabolism. They are, therefore, crucial for converting incoming substances (food, water, air) into energy in the cells.

TEST TYPE:     venous blood, chemistry

TEST OF:       blood, metabolism

TEST FOR:      level in blood

HOW OFTEN:     with symptoms

## estriol

DESCRIPTION: Hormone produced by the placenta during pregnancy. As the placenta grows, the level of estriol rises. This is thought to indicate normal, healthy development of the fetus.

Your lab sheet or technician may refer to a "triple test." This is an initial screen for fetal abnormalities and consists of **AFP**, unconjugated **estriol**, and **hCG**.

TEST TYPE:     plasma (from venous blood), chemistry

TEST OF:       placenta

TEST FOR:      level in blood

HOW OFTEN:     regularly with a high-risk pregnancy

NORMAL:          steady, even rise throughout pregnancy:

| | |
|---|---|
| 14 weeks | 0.53 ng/ml |
| 15 weeks | 0.66 ng/ml |
| 16 weeks | 0.83 ng/ml |
| 17 weeks | 1.05 ng/ml |
| 18 weeks | 1.31 ng/ml |
| 19 weeks | 1.65 ng/ml |
| 20 weeks | 2.08 ng/ml |
| 21 weeks | 2.61 ng/ml |

*Consult values given by your lab.*

HIGH:          multiple fetuses

LOW (drop in level or failure to rise): adrenal gland problem in fetus, anemia, diabetes, hypertension in the mother, kidney disease, liver disease, malnutrition, placental disorder (which may put the fetus at risk)

COMMENTS: Usually estriol is measured in the urine, but the blood test is available when needed.

## estrogens
### (estriol, estrone, estradiol)

DESCRIPTION: Hormones (female sex hormones, which means these are the substances that help produce female sexual characteristics) produced primarily in the ovaries but also in the placenta during pregnancy. Small amounts are produced by the adrenal glands and testicles. In women, levels vary with the menstrual cycle.

TEST TYPE:     venous blood, chemistry

TEST OF:       ovaries (gonadal function)

TEST FOR:      level in blood

HOW OFTEN:     with symptoms of sexual dysfunction or infertility

NORMAL:
- 12 - 115 pg/ml in men
- 24 -394 pg/ml first 2 weeks of menstrual cycle
  50 - 437 pg/ml at ovulation
  4 - 25 pg/ml during menses
  up to 31,000 pg/ml during pregnancy
  less than 40 pg/ml after menopause
- 3 - 10 pg/ml in children under age 6. *Consult range given by your lab.*

HIGH:          adrenal gland overactivity, liver disease, ovarian tumor, pituitary gland overactivity

LOW:           ovarian failure, pituitary gland underactivity

FALSE LOW:     <u>environment</u>: stress: athletic training and competition, dieting (severely reduced intake of calories)

FALSE RESULTS (HIGH or LOW):

<u>drugs</u>: antibiotics (ampicillin, tetracycline), birth control pills, hormones (estrogens, progesterone, cortisol), laxatives (cascara, senna), tranquilizers (meprobamate, phenothiazines), urinary tract medication (hydrochlorothiazide, phenazopyridine hydrochloride)

## ferritin
### (blood ferritin)

DESCRIPTION:  Protein which binds to iron thereby providing storage of iron for the body.

TEST TYPE:  venous blood, chemistry

TEST OF:  liver

TEST FOR:  iron storage

HOW OFTEN:  suspected deficiency

NORMAL:
- 15 - 350 ng/ml for men
- 12 - 204 ng/ml for women
- 7 - 600 ng/ml for children depending on age:
  7 - 140 ng/ml  age 6 months to 15 years
  200 - 600 ng/ml infants aged 1 month
  25 - 200 ng/ml newborns

*Consult the ranges given by your lab.*

HIGH:  chronic anemia (from defective red blood cells), Hodgkin's disease, infection, iron overload (too much iron deposited into body tissue), kidney disease, infection, inflammation, leukemia, liver disease

FALSE HIGH:  <u>medical</u>: recent blood transfusion

LOW:  chronic anemia (from iron deficiency)

## fetal monitoring

See individual tests in **boldface**:

- **AFP\***
- **estriol\***
- **hCG\***
- *lecithin/sphingolmyelin* ratio (expect maturity after 36 weeks gestation with l/s ratio over 2.5)
- prenatal panel: **blood type**, **Rh type**, **CBC**, indirect Coombs, hepatitis B surface antigen, rubella virus IgG antibody, rapid plasma reagin (RPR)

DESCRIPTION: *AFP, estriol and hCG were used in a 1994 study instead of *amniocentesis* as a screen for Down syndrome. Unusually high levels of all three predicted the syndrome in 89% of the test cases (as opposed to 100% accuracy with amniocentesis which carries the risk of miscarriage). Normal pregnancies were misidentified as abnormal in 25% of the cases. (*The New England Journal of Medicine* as reported by the *New York Times* April 24, 1994, page 27.)

## fibrinogen
### (plasma fibrinogen)

OTHER NAMES: Factor I

DESCRIPTION: The body responds quickly to injury. Whether an invisible (to us) break in the wall of a blood vessel or a scratch on our skin, an alarm goes out to plug the hole. Fibrinogen is a protein made in the liver which (along with *thrombin*, an enzyme made in the blood at the time of injury) becomes solid to form a blood clot or, more precisely, a *fibrin clot.*

TEST TYPE:        venous blood, chemistry

TEST OF:          liver

TEST FOR:         level in blood

HOW OFTEN:        with symptoms

NORMAL:           75 - 500 mg/dl. *Consult the range given on your lab sheet.*

HIGH:             cancer (kidney, stomach, breast), severe infection, vitamin K deficiency

LOW:              cancer (bone, prostate, pancreatic, lung), inherited blood disorders, liver disease, complications/ injury in childbirth, vitamin B deficiency

COMMENTS: Fibrinogen is removed from the blood (by allowing the blood to clot) before measuring **albumin** and **globulin** levels and is not included in total **protein** levels. Formation of the clot involves the conversion of **fibrinogen** to fibrin. A screening test to identify problems with conversion is the *thrombin time* test. Generally, if you are actively bleeding, ill or have an infection, or have received a blood transfusion within 4 weeks this test will not be given.

**fluoride**, see **poisoning**, page 148.

## folic acid

### (serum folate)

OTHER NAMES: folates (related compounds), pteroylglutamic acid, folacin

DESCRIPTION: A water-soluble vitamin not produced in the body, but essential for the body's health. With vitamin $B_{12}$, it influences red cell production, body growth and the formation of genes. *Folic acid* itself cannot be used until it is broken down into *folates* and absorbed by the small intestine. Once in the bloodstream, it is quickly absorbed by tissue.

Because it is used so quickly and only small amounts are stored in the liver, eating the right food every day is important, particularly liver, kidney, yeast, fruits, leafy vegetables, eggs and milk. Given its role in the production of genes, the demand for folic acid in pregnancy is greatly increased.

TEST TYPE:     venous blood, chemistry

TEST OF:     liver

TEST FOR:     level in blood

## folic acid (cont.)

HOW OFTEN:     suspected deficiency

NORMAL:        2 - 25 ng/ml. *Consult the range given by your lab.*

HIGH:          non-toxic in high doses, high levels can indicate you are eating too many folic acid-rich foods, taking too many supplements or you have a deficiency of vitamin $B_{12}$

LOW:           alcoholism, anemia, blood disease, poor diet, intestinal malabsorption, overactive thyroid

FALSE LOW:

- <u>diet</u>: too few folic acid-rich foods eaten, vitamin C deficiency
- <u>drugs</u>: cancer drugs, birth control pills, epilepsy medication (e.g., Dilantin)
- <u>environment</u>: pregnancy

COMMENTS:   Because serum folate levels change so quickly (reflecting diet and absorption), there is another test, *RBC folic acid*, which takes advantage of the fact that folate levels in red blood cells remain fairly constant and can be measured.  Normal levels fall below 95 ng/ml of RBCs.

**food poisoning**, see **poisoning**, page 148.
**fungicides**, see **poisoning**, page 149.

## galactose transferase
### (galactosemia screening)

OTHER NAMES: GALT, glactose-1-phosphate uridylic
transferase

DESCRIPTION: An enzyme which breaks down the sugar *galactose* (found in milk, sugar beets and seaweed). Without the enzyme, the sugar can cause considerable damage -- known as *galactosemia* -- to the eyes, kidney, liver and body tissue.

Galactosemia is hereditary and recessive: a child must receive an abnormal gene from both parents. Hence any parent can be a "carrier" (see LOW values below) without manifesting symptoms.

TEST TYPE: capillary blood (from heel) or cord blood (in newborns), venous blood (in adults), chemistry

TEST OF: metabolism

TEST FOR: level of amino acid

HOW OFTEN: at birth

NORMAL:
- **qualitative**: negative
- **quantitative**: 18.5 - 28.5 IU/gram of hemoglobin *Your lab sheet will say which type of test was used.*

POSITIVE: transferase deficiency

**galactose transferase** (cont.)

LOW:             less than 5 IU/g: galactosemia
                 5 - 18.5 IU/g: carrier state

COMMENTS: This is one of the tests considered mandatory in most states for newborns. If detected, organ damage can be avoided by a special diet.

**gamma globulin,** see **globulin** (page 80) and **immunoglobulins** (page 101) tests.

## GGT

**(gamma glutamyl transferase, gamma GT)**

## GGTP

**(gamma glutamyl transpeptidase, gamma GTP)**

DESCRIPTION: Enzymes produced by the liver which help to make the liver function as it should, breaking down, storing and transporting nutrients. (For example, GGT helps to transfer amino acids across cell membranes.)

TEST TYPE:       venous blood, chemistry

TEST OF:         liver

TEST FOR:        level in blood

HOW OFTEN:       with symptoms of liver damage

NORMAL:

**GGT**
- 0 - 45 U/l (men will have slightly higher levels)
- 0 - 75 U/l for men and women over age 64
- 0 - 270 U/l newborns to 6 days old
  0-120 U/l infants to age 2
  at age 12 adult levels are reached

**GGTP**
- 0 - 45 U/l for men
- 0 - 30 U/l for women
  Some labs report using the range 2-65 U/l without gender distinction. *Consult ranges given by your lab.*

HIGH:

alcoholism, liver disease/damage/tumors
**GGT**: also: brain tumor, epilepsy, jaundice, kidney disease, disorder of the pancreas

FALSE HIGH:

- diet: simple carbohydrates
- drugs: alcohol, pain medication (acetaminophen)

COMMENTS:   Both tests are used by insurance companies as indicators of alcoholism.
  GGT may increase 5 to 10 days after an acute heart attack.

# GHb

## (glycohemoglobin)

OTHER NAMES: total fasting hemoglobin test, glycosylated hemoglobin, $HgA_1$, $HgA_{1a-c}$. These terms are not synonymous. GHb, $HgA_1$ and $HgA_{1C}$ are different substances, requiring different laboratory procedures for measurement.

DESCRIPTION: This test is for diabetics. Instead of measuring your level of **insulin** or **glucose**, it measures how many hemoglobin molecules have sugar attached. Hemoglobin (**Hgb**) is part of a red blood cell so will show blood sugar activity of the preceding 6 to 8 weeks (the life cycle of a red blood cell). The **glucose tolerance test** only shows activity at the time of the test.

TEST TYPE: venous blood, chemistry

TEST OF: metabolism

TEST FOR: level in blood

HOW OFTEN: to monitor diabetes therapy

NORMAL:
- GHb    4.5% - 8 %
- $HgA_{1C}$    3% - 6% (about 75% of which is GHb)
- $HgA_1$    5.5% - 8.5% (about 18% of which is GHb; measurement can be affected by the presence of hemoglobin variants, page 92)

HIGH:              uncontrolled diabetes, inadequate treatment

FALSE HIGH/LOW: laboratory carelessness, failure to measure all forms of GHb, ethnic variations of hemoglobin that alter $HgA_{1C}$ results, high lipid level

## globulin
### (serum globulin)

DESCRIPTION:  Globulin is protein that circulates in the blood filling two different functions.  Some types act as a taxi service, transporting substances through the bloodstream, as does the protein **albumin**. These are the *alpha* and *beta* globulins, and are made in the liver. For example, *ceruloplasmin* is an $alpha_2$-globulin which carries most of the copper in the blood. *Transferrin* is a beta-globulin which binds and transports dietary iron.

Another type, the *gamma* globulins, are made in the immune system and patrol the blood looking for invaders.  They act, then, as immediate protection for the carrier proteins which might encounter disease-causing organisms in the blood.

A specialized test -- "serum protein electrophoresis" -- can measure the amount of each in the blood.  Together their levels in the blood make up the globulin level.  The globulin level is then used to calculate the level of total **protein** in the blood.

TEST TYPE:    venous blood, chemistry

TEST OF:      liver, immune response

TEST FOR:     level in blood

HOW OFTEN:    with symptoms

**globulin** (cont.)

NORMAL:

- 1.3 - 4.2 gm/dl for adults (over age 12)
  **alpha₁**  2.5% - 5% of total (0.1 - 0.4 gm/dl)
  **alpha₂**  7% - 15% of total (0.5 - 1 gm/dl)
  **beta**  8% - 14% of total (0.7 - 1.2 gm/dl)
  **gamma**  12% - 22% of total (0.5 - 1.6 gm/dl);
  see page 102 for levels of specific gammas
- 1.1 - 3.5 gm/dl for children. *Consult range given by your lab.*

HIGH:  cancer, chronic infections (including syphilis, tuberculosis), collagen diseases, diabetes, Hodgkin's disease, lupus, rheumatoid arthritis

FALSE HIGH:  medical tests: BSP (see page 214) within 48 hours before blood test

LOW:  blood disorder, kidney disease, liver dysfunction

## glucose

**(serum glucose)**

OTHER NAMES: dextrose, random blood sugar (RBS), fasting blood sugar, 2-hour postprandial blood sugar, fasting plasma glucose test

DESCRIPTION: *Glucose* is a form of sugar and is an essential by-product of carbohydrate digestion. When there is plenty of oxygen in the body's cells, glucose is broken down by oxidation (turning into water and carbon dioxide).

It is an important component of blood and is used as an immediate source of energy or stored as fat for later use. The body uses **insulin** to keep blood levels of glucose within the normal range.

Susceptibility to high values (and the associated diseases) is greater in those of Hispanic, African, native American or Japanese descent. Age also increases susceptibility as normal levels steadily increase after age 50.

TEST TYPE:    venous blood, chemistry

TEST OF:    liver, pancreas

TEST FOR:    level in blood

HOW OFTEN:    regular physical exam; suspected diabetes

NORMAL:    *Fasting* (12 hours)
- 70 - 125 mg/dl
  *Postprandial*
- 70-190 1 hour after eating
- 70 - 150 mg/dl, 2 hrs after eating
- 20 - 80 mg/dl in newborns after 1 hour

*Consult ranges given by your lab.*

HIGH:    brain tumor, carbon monoxide poisoning, central nervous system disease, Cushing's syndrome, diabetes, high blood pressure, infectious disease, kidney disorder, chronic liver disease, overactive endocrine glands, pancreatitis

**glucose** (cont.)

FALSE HIGH:

- <u>diet</u>: food containing arginine: brown rice, carob, chocolate, gelatin, oatmeal, popcorn, raisins, sesame seeds
- <u>drugs</u>: anesthesia, antibiotics, antipsychotics, asthma medication, birth control pills, blood pressure medication, diuretics, epilepsy medication, hormones, laxatives, poison neutralizer, steroids, vitamin B
- <u>environment</u>: large food intake prior to test, obesity, pregnancy, recent acute illness, exercise prior to test, smoking

LOW: adrenal insufficiency, inability to store sugar, liver disease, malabsorption, pancreatic disease, underactive pituitary gland, starvation

FALSE LOW:

- <u>diet</u>: poor nutrition
- <u>drugs</u>: alcohol, antidepressants (MAO inhibitors), heart medication (beta blockers), insulin
- <u>environment</u>: dehydration, exercise, exposure to the cold, fever

COMMENTS: This may be one of the blood chemistry values used to determine your acceptability for insurance (by checking for the presence of diabetes). See also the **GHb** test, page 79.

**glycohemoglobin.** See **GHb** test, page 79.
**gold**, see **poisoning**, page 149.

## GTT

### (glucose tolerance test)

DESCRIPTION: Used for diagnosing diabetes, there are actually several types of glucose tolerance tests as well as disagreement about interpreting the results.

The *oral glucose tolerance test* (OGTT) measures your body's tolerance to a large and concentrated dose of sugar over a 3- to 6-hour period. To get the best results, several days before the test include lots of carbohydrates (pasta, bread) in your diet. You will then be asked to fast from midnight the night before coming to the lab for the test. At the lab, blood and urine samples are taken, you are given a concentrated sugar solution to drink, and additional samples are taken at regular intervals. You should drink lots of water during the test (which helps the body break down the sugar). Also, don't smoke, use coffee or alcohol, or exercise strenuously for 8 hours before the test and during the test.

A *gestational glucose tolerance test* might be given to pregnant women between the 24th and 28th weeks of gestation. One test is similar to the above: several samples are drawn after fasting and drinking a slightly more concentrated glucose solution. Another test does not require fasting and only one sample is taken after drinking a less concentrated glucose solution.

A *fasting plasma glucose test* measures plasma glucose levels after a 12- to 14-hour fast. A *2-hour postprandial plasma glucose test* measures the level after a high-carbohydrate meal.

TEST TYPE:      venous blood, chemistry

TEST OF:        liver, pancreas

## GTT (cont.)

TEST FOR:        level in blood

HOW OFTEN:    suspected diabetes

NORMAL:         *fasting*
- 70 -120 mg/dl plasma
- 60 - 100 mg/dl whole blood

*1-hour after dose*
- 160 - 180 mg/dl (30-60 min)
- 70-190 mg/dl, gestational 1 hr,

*2-hours after dose*
- fasting level
- 70-165 mg/dl, gestational

*3-hours after dose*
- fasting level
- 70-145 mg/dl, gestational

*2-hour postprandial plasma glucose*
- below 145 mg/dl (higher over age 50)

LOW:               adrenal insufficiency (Addison's disease), Cushing's disease, central nervous system lesions, diabetes, pituitary underactivity, thyroid underactivity

COMMENTS: There is a similar test, *lactose tolerance test*, which measures blood sugar levels after drinking a dose of lactose (a form of sugar found in milk). This test collects 3 blood samples over a 2 hour period and asks for a stool sample 5 hours after taking the lactose.

## hCG
### (human chorionic gonadotropin)

OTHER NAMES: pregnancy test; some lab sheets say "HCG" -- it's the same thing (see the explanation on page 93)

DESCRIPTION: Hormone produced by the placenta during pregnancy. Home pregnancy tests test urine for the hormone which can start being detected 10 days after a missed menstrual period.

The blood test can detect the hormone earlier, as soon as 7 days after conception. There are two types of blood tests. Your lab sheet should say which test was used: a "positive" or "negative" result means that a *qualitative* serological test was used; an actual level reported means that a *quantitative* chemical measurement was made. Also used as a **tumor marker** for cancer of the testes.

TEST TYPE:      venous blood, serology, chemistry

TEST OF:        presence in blood

TEST FOR:       pregnancy

HOW OFTEN:      4-5 days after delay of menstrual period

NORMAL:         **qualitative**: negative
                **quantitative**:
- below 2.5 IU/l     males
- below 5 IU/l       premenopausal females
  below 10 IU/l      postmenopausal
  below 500 IU/l     0-2 weeks of pregnancy
  100-5,000 IU/l     2-3 weeks of pregnancy

## hCG (cont.)

500-10,000 IU/l    3-4 weeks of pregnancy
1,000-200,000 IU/l    1-2 months
10,000-100,000 IU/l    2-3 months

HIGH:    pregnancy, tumor. Unusually high levels of hCG may suggest a multiple pregnancy (twins or more). In nonpregnant persons, test may be used to screen for certain types of cancer.

LOW:    If pregnancy has been confirmed, but the level of hCG does not rise, there may be some problem with the pregnancy (it may occur outside the uterus or miscarriage may be likely).

FALSE LOW:    environment: test performed too early in pregnancy. (However, the hormone can be produced by the body as soon as 24 hours after implantation. It becomes detectable within 7-10 days of conception.)

COMMENTS: Your lab sheet or technician may refer to a "triple test." This is an initial screen for fetal abnormalities and consists of **AFP**, unconjugated **estriol**, and **hCG**, performed ideally during the 15th or 16th week of gestation.

Not too long ago, pregnancy was determined by injecting urine into immature mice, immature rats, rabbits, a female tree toad or a male frog (of a particular species).  All of these animals have unique responses to the hCG hormone.  If the woman donating the urine were pregnant, particular reactions from these animals would confirm the pregnancy.

## HCT

### (hematocrit)

OTHER NAMES: packed cell volume (PCV)

DESCRIPTION: This test looks at the quality of the red cells in the blood. Specifically, it is an indirect measure of the volume occupied by red blood cells in a sample. A centrifuge separates particles in the blood from the liquid. Used to calculate RBC indices, MCV and MCHC (see pages 167-168) as well as to diagnose anemia..

TEST TYPE:       venous or capillary blood, hematology, CBC

TEST OF:          whole blood

TEST FOR:         volume

HOW OFTEN:    regular physical exam

NORMAL:
- 40 - 50% in men
- 35 - 47% in women
- 31 - 41% in children
  44 - 64% in newborns.
  *Consult ranges given by your lab.*

HIGH:               blood/bone marrow disorder (causing overproduction of red blood cells), spontaneous blood clotting, dehydration, lung disease

## HCT (cont.)

FALSE HIGH: <u>environment</u>: carbon monoxide exposure, high altitude, smoking, surgery, tourniquet left on too long during test

LOW: anemia, blood disease, heart failure, infection, liver or spleen disease, toxins, tumors

FALSE LOW: <u>nutrition</u>: folic acid deficiency, iron deficiency, vitamin $B_{12}$ deficiency

## HDL

### (high density lipoprotein)

DESCRIPTION: Lipoproteins are the compounds that allow (nonsoluable) fats to move through the bloodstream: a protein carries a lipid (fat) to wherever the fat is needed.

It is not surprising that fat might form deposits in the bloodstream or attach themselves to the blood vessel walls, since fat is not soluble in blood and will be attracted to other fat particles. As we all know, this will immediately affect the heart's ability to move blood around the body.

One of the protein carriers of fat is HDL, which seems to do more than just transport. It appears to pick up *excess* fat (**cholesterol**) in the bloodstream, thus helping to clear the arteries. (If you have trouble remembering that HDL is the "good" cholesterol, think of "high density" as "able to carry a lot.")

TEST TYPE: venous blood, chemistry, lipid panel

TEST OF: heart

TEST FOR:      level in blood

HOW OFTEN:   every 5 years

NORMAL:

- 30 - 55 mg/dl in men
- 45 - 65 mg/dl in women *Consult ranges given by your lab.*

HIGH:         The upper level of "normal" and above are thought to decrease the risk of heart attack (when the **cholesterol:HDL ratio** is lower than normal). Levels can be further increased (in healthy persons) by exercise, not smoking and maintaining a stable weight within reasonable bounds. Although in earlier editions *Common Blood Tests* reported that moderate alcohol consumption seemed to elevate HDL, this same consumption is now showing an increased risk for breast cancer. Please remember that if you do regularly have alcohol, DON'T take acetaminophen for pain relief.

           Poor health can also raise lipid levels: bile duct obstruction, diabetes, kidney disease, pancreas disease, thyroid underactivity. Rarely, a sharp increase in *alpha$_2$-high-density lipoprotein* will point to heart disease.

FALSE HIGH:   <u>environment</u>: ingestion of alcohol/food prior to test, pregnancy

**HDL** (cont.)

LOW:           The lower the level of HDL, the greater the risk of heart attack (when the **cholesterol:HDL ratio** is higher than normal).

**hematocrit**
See **HCT** test, page 88.

## hematology
### (blood cell study)

See individual tests:

- **CBC**
- **coagulation panel**
- **retic count**
- **sed rate**

DESCRIPTION: In the widest sense, hematology refers to all study of blood: its behavior, chemistry, diseases. But many lab sheets use a much narrower sense: the size, shape and other physical characteristics of the blood cells.

TEST TYPE:     venous blood

TEST OF:       blood cells

TEST FOR:     appearance and behavior of blood

HOW OFTEN:   regular physical exam

# Hgb

## (hemoglobin)

OTHER NAMES: Hb, Hg, hemoglobin concentration

DESCRIPTION: *Hemoglobin* consists of iron and protein and is the part of the red blood cell that makes possible the exchange of gases. It carries **oxygen** from the lungs to body tissue and helps to return **carbon dioxide** to the lungs to be exhaled.

In the average person, there are three components of hemoglobin: A, $A_2$, and F. There can be further (genetic) variation in the protein portion of hemoglobin. Hence, you will see reference to hemoglobin S, C, E, etc. There are several hundred "variants." (See page 175 for a discussion of **hemoglobin S**.)

TEST TYPE:     capillary or venous blood, chemistry, CBC

TEST OF:      respiration

TEST FOR:     level in blood

HOW OFTEN:    regular physical exam

NORMAL:

- 12.4 - 18.0 g/dl in men
- 11.7 - 16.0 g/dl in women
- Except for high levels in newborns (which gradually drop to lowest level at age 2 months), readings in children are lower and increase with age:

    17-22 g/dl younger than 7 days
    15-20 g/dl 1 week

**Hgb** (cont.)
11-15 g/dl age 1 month
11-13 g/dl through childhood
**hemoglobin electrophoresis**
- hemoglobin A: greater than 95% of the above total
- hemoglobin $A_2$: 1.5% - 3.5% of total*
- hemoglobin F: less than 2%

HIGH:                dehydration, overproduction of red blood cells, *carrier of the genetic trait for *beta-thalassemia*

FALSE HIGH:    <u>environment</u>: tourniquet is left on too long

LOW:                anemia, fluid retention (edema), hemorrhage

COMMENTS: If you have diabetes, your doctor may monitor your level of *hemoglobin $A_{1C}$*. See the **GHb** test, page 79.

## hGH

### (human growth hormone)

OTHER NAMES: HGH, growth hormone, somatotrophic hormone; the use of the lower-case "h" in the name identifies the beginning word of the substance as "human" (as opposed to "high" in HDL or "hema" in HCT). Since HIV is only known with an upper-case "H," many have stopped using "h" in hGH and hCG.

DESCRIPTION: Secreted by the pituitary, hGH is the main regulator of human growth. Not surprisingly, as we age hGH seems to disappear. Even exercise stops stimulating the secretion of hGH around the age 30.

However, experimental use on a small group of elderly men produced such surprising results (e.g., increased muscle mass, increased elasticity of skin that it has been given much media attention, inducing adults to take hGH as a dietary supplement. This may not be wise; physicians caution against use at the present since having little or no hGH may be a protection against cancer.

TEST TYPE:     plasma (from venous blood), chemistry

TEST OF:     pituitary

TEST FOR:     level in blood

HOW OFTEN:     with symptoms; blood will be drawn on 2 con-
secutive days (between 6 am and 8 am)

NORMAL:     *First Sample*
- 0 - 8 ng/ml for males
- 0 - 10 ng/ml for females (higher due to effects of estrogren)
- 0 - 16 ng/ml for children
up to 40 ng/ml at birth
*Second Sample*
- 5 - 10 ng/ml for men
- 5 - 15 ng/ml for women

HIGH:     tumor of pituitary/hypothalamus, abnormal growth (*gigantism*, excessive height, in children and *acromegaly*, abnormal enlargement of the hands, feet, nose, jaw, in adolescents and adults), diabetes

**hGH** (cont.)

FALSE HIGH:

- <u>diet</u>: failure to fast
- <u>drugs</u>: amphetamines, estrogens (and all pituitary hormones), Parkinson's medication (levodopa), vitamin B
- <u>environment</u>: physical activity, excitement, radioactive scan within 1 week prior to test

FALSE NORMAL: <u>drugs</u>: hormones (corticosteroids), central nervous system depressants (phenothiazines: chlorpromazine) may suppress hGH

LOW: cancer, dwarfism, tumors

FALSE LOW:

- <u>diet</u>: failure to fast
- <u>drugs</u>: steroid medications
- <u>environment</u>: physical activity, excitement, radioactive scan within 1 week prior to test

## HIV
**(human immunodeficiency virus)**

DESCRIPTION: HIV is a virus which attacks white blood cells, specifically *lymphocytes*. It is hard to predict the behavior of the virus: it can remain dormant in you but be passed to others, it can attack a limited number of lymphocytes which means that you still have some defense against disease, or it can destroy nearly all your lymphocytes at which time a diagnosis of **AIDS** will probably be made (see page 11).

Two **antibody** tests are most commonly used for diagnosis: **ELISA** and **Western blot**. The ELISA is usually preferred for the initial screening: it is fairly simple and inexpensive. Western blot requires interpretation by a lab technician.

They are frequently used together in an "ELISA/WB package" because there is such a high rate of false positives with ELISA. After 2 positive ELISA's, a Western blot is given. If the WB is positive, another is given with a fresh blood sample. This procedure yields a very accurate result -- 0.0007% chance of error. See the *New England Journal of Medicine*, volume 319 (1988), page 961, for the study.

TEST TYPE:      venous blood, serology

TEST OF:        immune system

TEST FOR:       presence of antibody in blood

HOW OFTEN:      with symptoms or exposure

NORMAL:         negative: the following are test names that might appear on your lab sheet and the normal values for each

- **HIV-1 antibody confirmation by Western blot** p24, gp41, and gp120/160 are viral proteins (antigens); if no antibodies to these proteins are present in the blood sample, the sample is said to be "nonreactive"
- **HIV-1 antibody screen** = nonreactive
- **HIV-1 P24 antigen** = none detected. Antigens are detectable for a short period after infection and usually become undetectable after the appearance of antibodies to HIV-1. As the disease progresses,

**HIV** (cont.)

HIV-1 antigens usually become detectable again. High levels accompany AIDS symptoms and a low CD4 count, and suggest a poor prognosis.

- **HIV-1 proviral DNA in mononuclear cells (by PCR)** = none detected. A "provirus" is the DNA that HIV actually inserts into your cells if you become infected. "Mononuclear cells" are B-cells (having one nucleus, hence the name) duplicated in the lab to provide the best medium for testing. PCR (page 218) is a procedure which produces copies of a DNA segment to make evaluation of a blood sample easier.
- **Human T lymphocyte virus-1 antibody by EIA** = nonreactive
- **Immunocompetency panel**: absolute CD3, CD4, CD8, CD19 and cells in percent; helper to suppressor ratio, lymphocyte count, **WBC** count

IF YOU TEST POSITIVE:

The term "HIV" is being used to identify the disease as well as the virus, at least in the pre-AIDS stages. The Centers for Disease Control & Prevention in Atlanta suggests the following guideline for diagnosis.

### HIV asymptomatic

- you test positive for HIV
- your CD4+ T-lymphocyte count is above 500 mm$^3$ or at least 29% of the total lymphocyte count (see page 203)
- possible acute or primary HIV infection (an episode of flu-like illness sometimes called *HIV mononucleosis*) or *persistent generalized lymphadenopathy* (PGL, which means any disease of the lymph nodes). **Even though you may not be ill, you can still pass the virus to someone else.**

### HIV symptomatic

- you test positive for HIV
- your CD4+ T-lymphocyte is between 200 and 499 mm$^3$ or between 14% and 28% of the total lymphocyte count
- you have one or more AIDS-indicating conditions

At this stage, the virus is destroying a limited number of lymphocytes and there is still some defense against disease. However, the immune system is deteriorating. (Formerly, this stage was called "AIDS-related complex" or ARC.)

In children under 13, this category is further separated into **Mildly Symptomatic** and **Moderately Symptomatic**. In fact, the clinical diagnoses for children are somewhat different than those for adults and adolescents.

### AIDS

- you test positive for HIV
- your CD4+ T-lymphocyte count falls below 200 mm$^3$ or less than 14% of the total lymphocyte count
- you have one or more AIDS-indicating conditions, including *opportunistic* infections (see page 11)

FALSE POSITIVE:

- <u>environment</u>: defective test kit, damaged blood sample (blood chemistry can change with a change in temperature)
- <u>medical conditions</u>: alcoholism, connective tissue disease (such as lupus and arthritis), hemophilia, kidney disease requiring dialysis

COMMENTS: The virus does not behave like flu viruses, for example, which spread rapidly through the air or through casual contact. HIV is difficult to transmit. It passes from one person to another only in blood, semen and vaginal fluids. Even then, it must get into the *bloodstream* of the exposed person. For that reason, it is not usually transmitted through saliva, urine or other bodily fluids, even though the virus may be present. (*AIDS and the Mouth*, pp. 70-71, see *Bibliography*, page 224) It cannot travel through the air, through fluids (such as a swimming pool) or through food.

The tests mentioned above are all for HIV-1. There is, however, another strain -- HIV-2. Separate tests are required.

Not surprisingly, the behavior of HIV is affected by the presence of other diseases (as well as affecting the course of other diseases). Where there is simultaneous infection with tuberculosis or hepatitis, for example, HIV flourishes and the likelihood of AIDS increases. Conversely, TB will be more likely to develop into active infection in the presence of HIV.

Nor do HIV antibodies (found by the ELISA and Western blot tests) offer protection against disease as antibodies are supposed to.

## hormones

See individual tests (in **boldface**):
  *adrenal glands*

- **aldosterone**
- **cortisol** (corticosteroid)

  *kidney*

- angiotensin
- erythropoietin
- **renin**

  *pancreas*

- glucagon
- **insulin**

*pituitary gland*
- beta-melanocyte-stimulating hormone [to skin]
- corticotropin [to adrenal glands]
- endorphins [to brain]
- enkephalins [to brain]
- follicle-stimulating hormone (FSH) [to gonads]
- **hCG**
- **hGH** [to muscles and bones]
- luteinizing hormone (LH) [to gonads]
- oxytocin [to uterus and mammary glands]
- prolactin [to mammary glands]
- thyroid-stimulating hormone (TSH) [to thyroid]
- vasopressin (ADH) [to kidney]

*gonads:*
*ovaries*

- **estrogen**
- progesterone

*testes*

- **testosterone**

*thyroid glands*
- thyroid hormones **T₃, T₄**

   *parathyroid glands*
- parathyroid hormone

DESCRIPTION: *Hormones* are among the most powerful substances in the blood. They are secreted by glands: some regulate the activity of the glands themselves, others are sent to the body's organs to maintain a chemical balance. For example, hormones change the activity of key genes by either speeding up or suppressing their mechanism. This is why hormone therapy is so controversial -- its effects are far-reaching throughout the body. Estrogen replacement in menopausal women or human growth hormone used as an anti-

**hormones** (cont.)

aging drug, for two examples, may relieve a single symptom but at the same time the hormone is visiting all its other usual sites and stimulating changes wherever it goes.

**human chorionic gonadotropin**, see hCG test, page 86.

## immunoglobulins

OTHER NAMES: gamma globulins, Ig, antibodies

DESCRIPTION: *Immunoglobulins* are a type of white blood cell made from B lymphocytes, see page 207. These B cells circulate in the blood and create antibodies which destroy disease-causing organisms.

There are 5 types of immunoglobulins: **IgG** ("immunoglobulin G") attacks any foreign material, usually viruses, and will attack some bacteria, fungi, and toxins as a secondary response after IgM. It is the only immunoglobulin that crosses the placenta.

**IgA** responds more particularly to bacteria and viruses and protects the mucous membranes in the respiratory and GI tracts against invasion by microorganisms. It also activates the complement system.

**IgM** responds to infections and is the first antibody to appear. It produces antibodies against rheumatoid factors and gram-negative organisms, forms the ABO blood group, and helps to activate the complement system.

**IgE** is involved with allergic reactions and **IgD** is still not well understood but is present in some infections and absent in some hereditary deficiencies.

TEST TYPE:        venous blood, serology

TEST OF:     blood, immune response

TEST FOR:    level in blood

HOW OFTEN:  with symptoms

NORMAL:

**IgG** 5.0 - 20 mg/ml (about 75% of total)
**IgA** 0.3 - 4.0 mg/ml (about 15% of total)
**IgM** 0.2 - 2.0 mg/ml (about 5-7% of total)
**IgE** 0.001 - 0.01 mg/ml (2% or less of total)
**IgD** 1% or less of total.
These are adult values. Values in children are age-dependent. *Consult ranges given by your lab.*

HIGH:

**IgG**: IgG myeloma (a type of cancer), liver disease (e.g., hepatitis), lupus, pulmonary tuberculosis, rheumatoid arthritis, inflammation, autoimmune diseases
**IgA**: IgA myeloma, liver disease (e.g., hepatitis), lupus, rheumatoid arthritis, gastrointestinal infection, malabsorption
**IgM**: type 1 selective IgG and IgA deficiency, blood disease, kidney disease, liver disease (cirrhosis, hepatitis) lupus, rheumatoid arthritis, mononucleosis

**immunoglobulins** (cont.)

IgE: allergies, atopic skin disease (e.g., eczema), parasitic infestation, hay fever, asthma, anaphylactic shock, IgE myeloma
IgD: chronic infections, connective tissue disorders, some liver disease, IgD myeloma

FALSE HIGH: <u>drugs</u>: regular consumption of alcohol, methadone, or narcotics, estrogen therapy

LOW: **IgG**: selective IgG deficiency, AIDS, IgA myeloma, kidney disease
**IgA**: selective IgA deficiency, kidney disease
**IgM**: selective IgM deficiency, AIDS,
**IgD**: AIDS, hereditary deficiency syndromes

FALSE LOW:

- <u>drugs</u>: chemotherapy drugs (bacille Calmette-Guerin vaccine, methotrexate), epilepsy medication (phenytoin), hormones (methylprednisolone in high doses)
- <u>medical</u>: radiation therapy, chemotherapy

COMMENTS: Some immunoglobulins either destroy or react with the cell nucleus, hence they are known as *antinuclear antibodies.*
**IgG** can be further isolated into 4 subclasses in order to diagnose immunoglobulin deficiencies. It may also be used to help diagnose children with recurring infections. See *Specialized Blood Tests.*

**in phos** (inorganic phosphorus)
See **phos** test, page 133.

**indirect bili**
See **bilirubin** test, page 34.

## infertility studies
### (gonadal function)

See individual tests:

- **estrogens**
- **hCG** (human chorionic gonadotropin)
- **testosterone**

DESCRIPTION: Although testing for hormone levels is more specialized than screening for normal health, testing for fertility is becoming quite common. *Gonads* are specifically the testicles (in men) and ovaries (in women). Both (with the adrenal glands) produce **estrogens** and **testosterone**, which are responsible for the production of fertile eggs and sperm.

**insecticides**
See **poisoning** (organophosphates), page 152

# insulin

## (serum insulin)

DESCRIPTION: It is insulin that allows glucose into cells to be fed. That is why, of course, it is so important.

Insulin is a hormone made by the pancreas (although the stomach can secrete small amounts) which regulates the metabolism and transport of various nutrients.

To test the level in your blood, you will be asked to fast for 12 hours before the test. A blood sample will be taken and then you will be given a certain amount of a sugar solution to drink. (This is similar to the glucose tolerance test on page 84, which will be ordered if these results are uncertain.) Your blood insulin will be measured every half hour and should return to normal after 4 hours.

TEST TYPE:      venous blood

TEST OF:        pancreas

TEST FOR:       level in blood

HOW OFTEN:      with symptoms

NORMAL:

- 2 - 30 μu/ml, fasting (12 hours)
- over 200 μu/ml, within an hour. *Consult range given by your lab*

HIGH:           abnormally enlarged bones, liver disease, pancreatic disease/tumor

FALSE HIGH:

- <u>drugs</u>: hormones
- <u>environment</u>: surgery, obesity

LOW:            diabetes, heart attack

FALSE LOW:
- <u>drugs</u>: hormone-suppressors
- <u>environment</u>: emotional stress, surgery

### insurance tests

*Blood sample* may be used to test for:
- **chemistry**
  - ➤ **cholesterol**
  - ➤ fructosamine or **glucose** (blood sugar)
  - ➤ **GGTP**
  - ➤ toxicology (presence of drugs):
    - ▪ beta blockers
    - ▪ cocaine
    - ▪ diuretic agents
    - ▪ hypoglycemics
    - ▪ nicotine
- **serology**
  - ➤ **HIV**
  - ➤ pregnancy **(hCG)**

*Urine sample* may be used to test for:
- chemistry
  - ➤ creatinine
  - ➤ glucose
  - ➤ nicotine
  - ➤ protein
- residue (of cells or casts)
- specific gravity

**iodine**, see **poisoning**, page 149.

# iron
## (serum iron, Fe)

DESCRIPTION: Iron is the active component of hemoglobin. Hemoglobin (**Hgb**) is the part of the red blood cell that makes possible the exchange of gases by carrying **oxygen** throughout the body and returning **carbon dioxide** to the lungs to be exhaled.

Iron is present in other compounds as well. After being absorbed in the intestine, it is broken down, stored and distributed to where it is needed. But at this point, it is carried in the blood by the protein **transferrin**. This test measures the iron bound to transferrin in the blood.

TEST TYPE: venous blood, chemistry

TEST OF: metabolism

TEST FOR: level in blood

HOW OFTEN: regular physical exam

NORMAL:
- 25 - 200 mcg/dl in adults
- 55 - 185 mcg/dl in children. *Consult the ranges given by your lab.*

HIGH: anemia from iron overload (too much iron deposited into body tissue), hepatitis; see page 149 for possible toxicity

FALSE HIGH: drugs: birth control pills

LOW: anemia (from iron deficiency)

FALSE LOW:
- <u>diet</u>: iron deficiency
- <u>environment</u>: pregnancy

COMMENTS: Some doctors will request an "iron studies" series of tests. In addition to **iron**, this will include the tests for **ferritin, TIBC** and RDW.

## kidney function tests

See individual tests:

- albumin
- BUN
- calcium
- chloride
- creatinine
- phosphorus
- potassium
- sodium

OTHER NAMES: renal function studies

DESCRIPTION: The function of the kidney is to filter blood, separating essential elements from waste products. It captures the fluid waste to send to the bladder where it will be excreted as urine.

Because the kidneys are extracting fluid from the body, they will have to replace the fluid (with the proper pH) in order to keep the blood's pressure, viscosity, and acid-base balance stable. This becomes a rather sophisticated juggling act. Albumin is the kidney's on-site representative in the blood, monitoring pressure, viscosity and volume; BUN (blood urea nitrogen) and creatinine are waste products; calcium, chloride, phosphorus, potassium and sodium are electrolytes responsible for creating the necessary pH.

TEST TYPE:      venous blood, chemistry

TEST OF:          kidney

TEST FOR:        level in blood

HOW OFTEN:     regular physical exam

# LD

### (lactic dehydrogenase)

DESCRIPTION: Heart enzyme, also found in other body tissues, which helps with metabolism. When cells are damaged, LD levels will increase. To find out where the damage is, *isoenzymes* can be isolated. Also used as a **tumor marker** to identify some cancers.

TEST TYPE:    venous blood, chemistry

TEST OF:    heart, liver

TEST FOR:    level in blood

HOW OFTEN:    with symptoms

NORMAL:    80 - 260 IU/l or
200 - 600 U/m. *Consult range given by your lab.* The extreme variation is due to different methods of testing used by labs.
$LD_1$ isoenzyme from the heart: **14-36%** of total
$LD_2$ isoenzyme from the red blood cells/kidney: **29-50%** of total
$LD_3$ isoenzyme from the lungs: **15-26%** of total
$LD_4$ isoenzyme from the liver: **2-16%** of total
$LD_5$ isoenzyme from the skeletal muscles **3-16%** of total

**LD** (cont.)

HIGH: anemia, cancer, heart attack, leukemia, liver disease, pulmonary embolism, tissue damage
$LD_1$ and $LD_2$ : cancer (leukemia, non-Hodgkin's lymphoma, Ewing's sarcoma, cancer of the testes)

FALSE HIGH: drugs: alcohol, anesthetics, aspirin, narcotics

FALSE LOW:
- drugs: ascorbic acid (vitamin C)
- environment: contamination of specimen by an oxalate (page 153)

COMMENTS: $LD_1$ is also known as *hydroxybutyric dehydrogenase* (HBD) which can be easier and cheaper to measure by itself than an electrophoresis of all the LD isoenzymes. It can't reliably distinguish between heart and liver cellular damage but can be useful in diagnosing heart attack. Serum values range from 114-290 U/l; ratio of serum LD to HBD varies from 1:2 - 1.6:1.

## LDL

### (low density lipoprotein, serum LDL cholesterol)

DESCRIPTION: Lipoproteins are the compounds that allow (nonsoluable) fats to move through the bloodstream: a protein carries a lipid (fat) to wherever the fat is needed. It seems to be LDL that actually delivers fat to the cells. (*Very low-density lipoproteins* -- **VLDLs** -- carry triglycerides to fat deposits.) LDL also seems to "deliver" excess cholesterol into the bloodstream, hence increasing the risk of heart attack.

Your lab may take the average of two tests to determine your level of LDL, 1 to 8 weeks apart. Each test actually consists of two additional readings: an initial measurement and a second measurement after a 12-hour fast. So if you think of a blood test as actually having the blood drawn, your LDL test might require 4 blood tests.

TEST TYPE:      venous blood, chemistry, lipid panel

TEST OF:        heart

TEST FOR:       level in blood

HOW OFTEN:      every 5 years

NORMAL:

- **LDL**
  below 110-130 (younger than 20)
  below 130-160 mg/dl (20+years old)
- **LDL:HDL ratio**: 3.2 - 3.5
- **VLDL**

| VLDL | men | women |
|---|---|---|
| ages 5-19 | 0-26 mg/dl | 1-24 mg/dl |
| 20's | 1-36 mg/dl | 2-29 mg/dl |
| 30's | 5-56 mg/dl | 1-36 mg/dl |
| 40's | 5-51 mg/dl | 5-41 mg/dl |
| 50's | 8-62 mg/dl | 2-49 mg/dl |
| 60's | 4-45 mg/dl | 1-41 mg/dl |
| 70+ | 0-38 mg/dl | 0-48 mg/dl |

*Consult ranges given by your lab.*

HIGH:           The upper level of "normal" and above are thought to increase the risk of heart attack (when the LDL:HDL ratio is higher than normal).

**LDL** (cont.)

FALSE HIGH:

- <u>diet</u>: eggs/brains in the 12-hour period before the test
- <u>drugs</u>: asthma medication, birth control pills (C-19 Progestin), corticosteroids, cortisone, diuretics (thiazides), epilepsy medication, male hormones (androgens), sedatives, vitamins A and D
- <u>environment</u>: absence of oxygen (high altitudes), pregnancy, rough handling of sample (resulting in damage to red blood cells), ingestion of alcohol/food prior to test, pregnancy

LOW:

The lower the level, the lower the risk of heart attack (when the LDL:HDL ratio is lower than normal). Disease conditions producing low levels include: AIDS, cancer, cerebral hemorrhage, chronic anemia infection, liver damage, malnutrition, thyroid overactivity

FALSE LOW:

- <u>drugs</u>: antibiotics, aspirin, female hormones (estrogens), vitamin $B_3$
- <u>environment</u>: fasting

COMMENTS: If you are a candidate for heart disease, your doctor may want to measure levels of *lipoprotein(a)*, a genetic relative of LDL which also helps identify risk.

It may be, then, that LDL can help diagnose the early and fatal heart disease causing the deaths of young athletes in good physical condition. Parents may want to ask their doctor for such a screen as their children pursue sports -- not because sports is a risk factor, but because early detection of a problem is now possible.

## lead

DESCRIPTION: A mineral that should never be in our bodies because it inhibits the production of hemoglobin (which carries oxygen). However, we do take in lead from the environment* (see COMMENTS on the next page). Industrial workers, people exposed to automobile exhaust fumes and children are at the greatest risk of building up toxic levels of lead.

Some lead is excreted by the kidneys. Most of the inorganic lead is incorporated into the red blood cells and ends up in the bones, teeth, liver and brain. Exposure to organic lead (e.g., *tetraethyl lead* used in leaded gasoline) is equally dangerous but confined to people who make, transport or otherwise handle these compounds.

TEST TYPE:    venous blood, chemistry

TEST OF:    blood

TEST FOR:    presence and level in blood

HOW OFTEN:    with symptoms

NORMAL:

- 0 - 30 mcg/dl in adults (this is the threshold set by OSHA, the Occupational Safety and Health Administration) or
  "free erythrocyte protoporphyrin" below 35 mcg/dl
- 0 - 25 mcg/dl in children
  below 10 mcg/dl for ages under 6
  below 25 mcg/dl for ages over 6. As the level reaches the upper limit, some doctors will begin

**lead** (cont.)

monitoring the level (testing regularly) and will ask for an investigation to determine how the lead is being ingested. *Consult ranges given by your lab.*

HIGH:  lead poisoning (also called *plumbism* because the Latin name for lead is "plumbum")

COMMENTS: Zinc protoprophyrin (ZPP) can also accumulate in red blood cells as a result of chronic lead absorption. If your lab measures this level, it should be below 70 mcg/dl.

*Uses of lead include soldering, paint pigments, storage batteries, ceramics, pesticides, plastics, alloys to make machine parts, ammunition, cosmetics, pottery making, and some medicines. Consequently, lead can be in the soil and water which is how some ends up in our food.

## lipase

**(serum lipase)**

OTHER NAMES: pancreatic lipase

DESCRIPTION: Digestive enzyme which breaks down fat. It is made in the pancreas and secreted into the upper portion of the intestine (the *duodenum*). There it converts triglycerides and other fats into fatty acids and glycerol. High values of any enzyme mean that it is leaking from the cells/tissues into the bloodstream (from injury or overproduction).

TEST TYPE:  venous blood, chemistry

TEST OF:      pancreas, endocrine glands

TEST FOR:     level in blood

HOW OFTEN:   with symptoms; after surgery

NORMAL:      0 - 110 U/dl
0 - 1.5 IU/ml or
0 - 0.08 mg/dl or
14 - 280 mIU/ml. *Consult range given by your lab.*

HIGH:         bile duct/ intestinal obstruction, kidney disease, liver disease, pancreatic disease*, ulcers (perforated)

FALSE HIGH:   <u>drugs</u>: diuretics, narcotics

COMMENTS:  *High levels of **amylase** (page 23) with high levels of lipase point to problems with the pancreas.

## lipid panel

### (analysis of blood fats)

See individual tests (in boldface); the other tests are also of lipids but are not included in *Common Blood Tests*:

- **cholesterol**
- fatty acids
- **HDL**
- ketones
- **LDL**
- phospholipid
- serum observation, see **blood smear**
- total lipids
- **triglycerides**

DESCRIPTION: Lipids are the fats carried through the bloodstream by proteins (as *lipoproteins*). See the list of transport proteins under **plasma**, page 137.

TEST TYPE:     venous blood, chemistry

TEST OF:        liver, heart

TEST FOR:       level in blood

HOW OFTEN:    regular physical exam

**lipoprotein phenotyping**
See **HDL** (page 89) and **LDL** (page 111).

**lipoprotein-cholesterol fractions**
See **HDL** (page 89) and **LDL** (page 111).

**lithium**
See **poisoning**, page 150.

## liver function tests

See individual tests (in boldface); the others also test for liver function but are not included in *Common Blood Tests*:

- **albumin***
- **alk phos*** (alkaline phosphatase)
- **ALT*** (SGPT)
- **ammonia**
- **AST*** (SGOT)
- **bilirubin*: direct, indirect, total**
- **cholesterol**
- **coagulation panel**
- **glucose**
- **LD** (lactate dehydrogenase)
- 5'-nucleotidase
- **pro time**
- SLAP (see COMMENTS on the next page)
- total **protein**

OTHER NAMES: *hepatic function panel*. Labs will offer a range of liver function panels (groups of tests done together). In the case of this panel, these seven tests are used. Your lab sheet will usually list the individual tests when a panel is ordered.

DESCRIPTION: The liver is part of the *gastrointestinal* (GI) system. It is the GI system that transforms what we eat into food for our cells and takes out the garbage (what we can't use). The liver, in particular, stores nutrients as starch (glucose) and fat (cholesterol), as well as storing vitamins and minerals.

The liver also helps to produce the protein cells found in the blood, the clotting "factors" (see **coagulation panel** and **pro time** tests), and the enzymes (**ALT, AST, LD**) which help diagnose damage to the heart muscle.

TEST TYPE:     venous blood, chemistry

TEST OF:       liver

TEST FOR:      level in blood

COMMENTS: *Serum leucine aminopeptidase* (SLAP) is another enzyme used in the metabolism of amino acids for absorption in the intestine. Its level should be 1 - 3 μmoles/hr/ml; increased values point to biliary tract, liver or pancreatic disease. This test is rarely used now.

## Lyme disease

DESCRIPTION: A multi-stage disease caused by a spirochete (another disease-causing germ) transmitted through a bite from a deer tick. The first test is an **ELISA**; if the results are indeterminate or positive, the more sensitive **Western blot** test will allow for better diagnosis.

TEST TYPE: venous blood, serology

TEST OF: blood

TEST FOR: presence of antibody

HOW OFTEN: with exposure (tick bite and rash)

NORMAL: negative

FALSE NEGATIVE: too early to have made antibodies

POSITIVE: presence of *Borrelia burgdorferi*

FALSE POSITIVE: presence of other spirochetes, rheumatoid factor; sample will be retested using more sensitive procedures

COMMENTS: The blood tests for Lyme disease are notoriously inaccurate, sometimes giving a negative test result even after the tick bite, "bulls eye" rash (*erythema chronicum migrans*, ECM) and subsequent symptoms have been confirmed.

Since the spirochete can live in the body long after the rash is gone, genetic testing has been successfully used to identify it in the joint fluid of patients with chronic arthritis. (*The New England Journal of*

*Medicine*, January 27, 1994, vol. 330, no. 4)

As this volume went to press, a new test was approved by the Food & Drug Administration which is claimed to have a higher degree of accuracy. You might want to inquire, if you have doubts about the results of your test, about which test kit was used by the lab or whether your sample was sent out to another lab.

**lymphocytes** (type of white blood cell).
See **WBC diff**, page 207.

# magnesium, Mg⁺⁺

DESCRIPTION: A mineral needed by the nerves and muscles of the body.  It also helps move small molecules across cell membranes.  Because it is (positively) charged, it is part of the electrolyte balance in the body's fluids.  Absorbed through the intestines and excreted through the kidneys and colon.

TEST TYPE:  venous blood, chemistry

TEST OF:  metabolism

TEST FOR:  level in blood

HOW OFTEN:  with symptoms

NORMAL:  1.2-3.0 mg/dl. *Consult range given by your lab.*

HIGH:  Addison's disease, adrenal gland underactivity, dehydration, heart attack, kidney failure; see page 150 for symptoms of toxicity

FALSE HIGH:  drugs: antacids, magnesium salts (milk of magnesia, Epsom salts) or supplements

LOW:  adrenal gland overactivity, alcoholism, burns, diarrhea, intestinal malabsorption, malnutrition, pancreas infection, thyroid gland (or parathyroid gland) overactivity

FALSE LOW:

- drugs: diuretics (thiazides, ethacrynic acid)
- medical treatment: long-term IV (tube) feeding
- nutrition: excessive calcium

### manganese

DESCRIPTION: a mineral that resembles iron, it helps to activate the enzymes that carry on the body's functions. Can be toxic (see page 150). Eaten in unrefined cereals, green leafy vegetable, nuts.

TEST TYPE:    venous blood, chemistry

TEST OF:    metabolism

TEST FOR:    level in blood

HOW OFTEN:    with symptoms

NORMAL:    0.04 - 1.4 mcg/dl

HIGH:    deterioration of central nervous system, edema (retaining water), liver disease, lung infection, manganese poisoning (see page 150)

FALSE HIGH:    <u>drugs</u>: manganese supplements

LOW:    epilepsy

**MCV** (Mean Cell Volume), **MCH** (Mean Cell Hemoglobin), **MCHC** (Mean Cell Hemoglobin). See **RBC indices**, page 167.

**mercury**
See **poisoning**, page 150.

**narcotics**
See **poisoning**, page 151.

## metabolic function

See individual tests:

| basic metabolic panel | comprehensive metabolic panel | |
| --- | --- | --- |
| **BUN** | **albumin (& a/g ratio)** | |
| **BUN/creatinine ratio** | **alk phos** | **AST** |
| **carbon dioxide** | **bilirubin** | **BUN** |
| **chloride** | **BUN/creat ratio** | **chloride** |
| **calcium creatinine** | **globulin** | **glucose** |
| **creatinine** | **potassium** | **protein** |
| **glucose** | **sodium** | |
| **potassium** | | |
| **sodium** | | |

DESCRIPTION: *Metabolism* is the activity of transforming nutrients (carbohydrates, fats, proteins, minerals, vitamins, water, oxygen) into energy or new material for the body. Since it involves all the chemical activities of the body, all of the blood tests provide information either directly or indirectly about the body's metabolic function.

The tests in the *basic metabolic panel* check the specific activities of carbohydrate metabolism, (**glucose, potassium**), protein metabolism (**BUN**), fluid balance (**chloride, sodium**), and waste disposal (**carbon dioxide, creatinine**).

TEST TYPE:     venous blood, chemistry

TEST OF:     metabolism

TEST FOR:     level of substance in blood

**monocytes**, see **WBC diff**, page 206.

**MPV** (Mean Platelet Volume), see **platelet evaluation**, page 139.

**narcotics**
See **poisoning**, page 151.

**neutrophils**
See **WBC diff**, page 204.

## newborn tests
### (neonatal screening)

| Often Mandatory | Optional |
|---|---|
| blood group | CBC |
| hemoglobin electrophoresis | galactosemia |
| HIV | retic count |
| PKU | TORCH |
| Rh factor | |
| sickle cell screening | |
| $T_4$ | |

**nickel**
See **poisoning**, page 151.

**nicotine**
See **poisoning**, page 151.

**NPN** (nonprotein nitrogen)
See **BUN**, page 39.

**organophosphates**
See **poisoning**, page 152.

## osmolality

### (serum osmolality)

DESCRIPTION: Measures the concentration of particles in the blood (*viscosity*). When the blood is too thick (or too thin), the pituitary gland sends a hormonal message to the kidney to slow down (or speed up) the excretion of water. This test might be useful, then, in the study of electrolyte and water balance.

Osmolality can also be calculated: your lab sheet will tell you which test was used. Levels of **sodium, glucose,** and urea nitrogen (**BUN**) are used for this calculation.

TEST TYPE:      venous blood, rheology

TEST OF:        pituitary gland, kidney, fluid balance

TEST FOR:       blood concentration

HOW OFTEN:      with symptoms

NORMAL:         274 - 305 milliosmols/kg. *Consult range given by your lab.*

HIGH:           dehydration, kidney disease, pituitary gland disease
FALSE HIGH:
- drugs: diuretics
- environment: loss of fluid due to heat or activity

LOW:            overhydration, pituitary disease

COMMENTS: Some laboratories give the *specific gravity* of the blood sample. This measures the density of the serum compared with pure water (1.000). Normal range is 1.025 - 1.029.

There is a specialized blood test for *osmotic fragility* which is a different test. This test measures the relative strength of the red blood cell walls and may be used to help diagnose a specific anemia.

**oxalates**
See **poisoning**, page 153.

### oxygen, $O_2$

DESCRIPTION: There are several types of measures of oxygen in the blood. *Oxygen content* tells the percentage of $O_2$ in the sample. *Oxygen capacity* predicts how much oxygen the blood *could* hold. *Oxygen saturation* combines the above values to indicate how much oxygen is available to the body. *Oxygen tension* (also called the *partial pressure of oxygen* or $pO_2$) measures the actual mass of oxygen in the blood.

TEST TYPE:     arterial and venous blood, chemistry

TEST OF:     respiration

TEST FOR:     level in blood

HOW OFTEN:     with symptoms

NORMAL:     *Oxygen content*
        15% - 23% for arterial blood
        10% - 16% for venous blood
     *Oxygen capacity*
        16% - 24% (varies with the amount of hemoglobin in the blood)

**oxygen** (cont.)
*Oxygen saturation*
  95% - 100% for arterial blood
  60% - 85% for venous blood
*Oxygen tension* or $pO_2$
  75 - 105 mm Hg.
*Consult ranges given by your lab.*

HIGH:    unlikely, although hyperventilating (panting) might well increase values

LOW:    asthma or emphysema, blood disease (e.g., too many red blood cells), lung disease, respiratory impairment
*Oxygen content*: when breathing is normal, suggests severe anemia, decreased blood volume, reduced oxygen-carrying capacity.

FALSE LOW:    environment: exercise

COMMENTS: A normal by-product of metabolism is *free radicals*, ionized oxygen $(O_2^-)$. Even in its non-ionized form, oxygen has a remarkable effect on whatever it comes into contact with (note the formation of rust on the surface of iron). The *ionized* form of oxygen is capable of doing considerable damage to cells and tissues in the body. Vitamins C and E are especially effective in neutralizing free radicals.

We associate the air we breathe with oxygen and the air we exhale with carbon dioxide. However, $^4/_5$'s of "air" is nitrogen. Shouldn't we be saturated with more nitrogen than anything else? Nitrogen dissolves easily in the body's fluids and becomes part of protein and nucleic acids. It only returns to gaseous form in the body if the atmospheric pressure drops (which is what gives "bends" to re-surfacing divers).

**pancreas function**
See **insulin** test, page 105.

## parathyroid function

See individual tests:

- **calcium**
- **phos**(phorus)

DESCRIPTION: As part of the endocrine system, the parathyroid gland produces the hormone, PTH (*parathyroid hormone*), which controls the electrolyte balance in the blood. The above tests tell how well PTH is doing its job.

TEST TYPE:       venous blood, chemistry

TEST OF:         parathyroid gland, kidney

TEST FOR:        level in blood

HOW OFTEN:       regular physical exam

**partial thromboplastin time**
See **PTT** test, page 165.

**PCBs**
See **poisoning**, page 153.

**PCP**
See **poisoning**, page 153.

# pH
## (potential [of] hydrogen [ions])

OTHER NAMES: [logarithmic] power of hydrogen

DESCRIPTION:  In order for us to exhale the carbon dioxide created by metabolism, most of the carbon dioxide entering the bloodstream breaks down into hydrogen ions (positively charged, acidic) and bicarbonate ions.  The hydrogen ions are picked up by the hemoglobin to carry back to the lungs.

The number of hydrogen ions in a solution defines whether the solution is "acid" or "alkaline" (*acid* or *base*, whether the solution is below or above the number 7 -- the number designated as "neutral").

Our blood, then, is slightly alkaline which means it carries a slightly negative charge.  It is within this very narrow range that we are healthy and our blood can do its best.  Having the proper **acid-base balance** means keeping within this range.

TEST TYPE:      arterial and venous blood

TEST OF:        kidney, respiration

TEST FOR:       the electrical charge of blood

HOW OFTEN:      with symptoms

NORMAL:
- 7.32 - 7.46 in adults
- 7.38 - 7.42 in children.  *Consult range given by your lab.*

HIGH:           blood is too alkaline: overactive adrenal function, coma, dehydration, buildup of carbon dioxide in the blood (respiratory alkalosis, for example; when someone hyperventilates or breathes too rapidly the resulting light-headedness is because the blood has become too alkaline; any overstimulation of the lungs can cause this)

FALSE HIGH:

- <u>drugs</u>: aspirin
- <u>environment</u>: fluid loss (from diarrhea, exercise, rapid breathing, sweating), oxygen deficiency (anxiety, high altitude), use of tourniquet may affect values

LOW:  blood is too acid: too much water in blood (which can be toxic), loss of carbon dioxide in the blood (respiratory acidosis, from emphysema or other lung disease), overstimulation of nervous system (muscle spasms, convulsions)

FALSE LOW:  <u>drugs</u>: antacids

COMMENTS: Some labs will test the **acid-base balance** of the blood in an **anion gap** test. An "anion" is a negatively charged particle. The results of the test should be the same as for **pH**, slightly alkaline.

Evaluated with the tests for **bicarbonate, carbon dioxide** and **oxygen**.

## phos, P
### (phosphorus, phosphates)

OTHER NAMES: inorganic phosphorus/phosphate ("in phos")

DESCRIPTION: *Phosphorus* is a mineral taken in from the food we eat, mainly dairy products, meat, egg yolks, legumes, nuts. In the blood, as in most things, it appears as electrolytes (specifically, "anions" with a negative charge). These *phosphate ions* help metabolism, maintain our **acid-base balance**, regulate **calcium** levels, and form bones (about 85% is stored in the bones as *calcium phosphate*); absorbed through the intestines and excreted by the kidneys.

TEST TYPE:       venous blood, chemistry

TEST OF:         parathyroid gland, acid-base balance

TEST FOR:        level of phosphate ions

HOW OFTEN:       regular physical exam

NORMAL:
- 2.3 - 4.7 mg/dl in adults
- 4.0 - 7.0 mg/dl in children. *Consult range given by your lab.*

HIGH:            bone disease, underactive parathyroid, overactive pituitary, kidney failure, diabetic acidosis, intestinal obstruction, toxicity (see page 154)

FALSE HIGH:

- <u>drugs</u>: blood thinner (anticoagulant), epilepsy medication, hormones, steroids
- <u>environment</u>: bone fracture, phosphorus or vitamin D excess, rough handling of specimen

LOW: alcoholism, calcium overload, kidney disease, malabsorption, malnutrition, overactive parathyroid, rickets

FALSE LOW:

- <u>drugs</u>: antacids, asthma medication (epinephrine), diabetes medication (insulin), diuretics, glaucoma medication
- <u>environment</u>: dehydration, IV (intravenous) solution, phosphorus or vitamin D deficiency in diet

COMMENTS: Level should be the inverse of **calcium** level (high when calcium is low, low when calcium is high).

## pituitary gland function

See individual test:        **hGH**

DESCRIPTION: As part of the endocrine system, the pituitary produces the hormones which prompt the other glands to produce their hormones. For example, the hormone **hGH** regulates growth which requires stimulating the thyroid gland.

TEST TYPE:        venous blood, chemistry

TEST OF:        pituitary gland

TEST FOR:        level in blood

HOW OFTEN:        regular physical exam


## PKU

### (phenylketonuria screening)

OTHER NAMES: Guthrie test, phenylalanine

DESCRIPTION: *Phenylalanine* is an amino acid essential to growth and nitrogen balance. If it accumulates in the blood (i.e., if not broken down properly by the body), the accumulation can cause mental retardation and abnormal development of the nervous system. This condition is called *phenylketonuria.*

TEST TYPE:        capillary blood (from heel), chemistry

TEST OF:        metabolism

TEST FOR:        level of amino acid

HOW OFTEN:       after birth, 24 hours after first milk; after 3-4 days
                 of milk or formula feeding

NORMAL:          0 - 4 mg/dl. Some labs require levels of less than
                 2 mg/dl. *Consult range given by your lab.*

FALSE NORMAL:
- drugs: antibiotics
- medical: presence of phenyllactic acid, phenyl-
  pyruvic acid

HIGH:            enzyme system malfunction, galactosemia (see
                 page 76), liver disease, PKU

COMMENTS: This is one of the tests considered mandatory in most
states for newborns. If detected, PKU can be avoided by a special diet.
There is a much less sensitive urine test available.

Higher incidence of PKU occurs in Caucasians, particularly those of
Irish or Scottish descent.

## plasma

DESCRIPTION: Plasma is the liquid part of the blood and consists of water (over 90%), proteins (about 7% by weight) and small amounts of fatty substances, inorganic substances, glucose, amino acids, vitamins, hormones.

*Plasma proteins* (sometimes called "carrier proteins") transport non-soluble substances through the blood.  See the tests for **albumin, globulin, TIBC,** and total **protein**.

*Plasma lipids* are fats which must be attached to a protein to move through the bloodstream.  In this form they are "lipoproteins."

*Glucose* is commonly known as "blood sugar" and is the form used to move carbohydrates and sugar from the diet through the blood to the body's tissues.

*Inorganic substances* include the electrolytes and trace minerals necessary for our health.  See the tests for **bicarbonate, calcium, chloride,** copper (page 146), **iron, potassium,** and **sodium**.

*Plasma hormones* all come from the endocrine system.  For the specific hormones in the blood, see the function tests for the **adrenal glands,** the **pancreas** and the **thyroid**.

NORMAL:  60% of our body weight: about $^2/_3$'s is contained in the fluid in the cells (*intracellular fluid*, ICF), the remaining $^1/_3$ is outside the cells (*extracellular fluid*, ECF -- some in the blood vessels).

COMMENTS: Fluid volume and how it is distributed throughout the body will be an indication of health.  In order to evaluate this, your doctor may order **arterial blood gases, electrolytes,** and **osmolality** tests.

## platelet evaluation

DESCRIPTION: *Platelets* are cell fragments produced by the bone marrow that assist in clotting. These fragments actually patch a hole or clump together to slow blood loss when you are injured. Often ordered with **PT** and **PTT** tests.

TEST TYPE:      capillary or venous blood, rheology

TEST OF:        clotting function of blood

TEST FOR:       platelet number and size, speed of clotting

HOW OFTEN:      when bleeding disorders are suspected; to verify proper clotting; prior to surgery

**platelet aggregation test:** used to measure how quickly the platelets in a blood sample clump together after an aggregating agent is added to the test tube.

NORMAL:         3-5 min. (following an 8-hour fast or elimination of fat from the diet). *May vary due to temperature or lab protocol. Use the range given on your lab sheet.*

SLOW:           various blood diseases including hemophilia

FALSE SLOW:     <u>drugs:</u> aspirin/aspirin compounds (need to be withheld for 14 days before the test), antihistamines, antiinflammatory drugs, tricyclic antidepressants

## platelet evaluation (cont.)

COMMENTS: Aspirin dilates (widens) blood vessels. This is why low dosage (80 mg daily or 325 mg every other day) is recommended for people who may be prone to blood clots in an artery or vein.

**platelet count** (thrombocyte count): Your lab sheet will show whether an *estimate* or an actual count was done. A **platelet estimate** is given as "low," "normal/average," or "increased."

NORMAL: 150,000 - 400,000 platelets/mm$^3$ *Consult range given by your lab.*

HIGH: anemia, arthritis, bleeding, blood cell disintegration, infection, inflammation, leukemia

FALSE HIGH:

- environment: exercise, pregnancy
- medical: removal of spleen
- nutrition: iron deficiency

LOW: anemia, bone marrow disease, cancer, infection, enlarged spleen

FALSE LOW:

- drugs: antibiotics, antiinflammatory medication, arthritis medication, diuretics (thiazides), heart beat regulator, sedatives, steroids
- nutrition: deficiency of folic acid or vitamin $B_{12}$

**mean platelet volume** (MPV): the measure of the average volume of a single platelet, to suggest whether they are of normal size. Young platelets are generally larger and will produce the best clotting.

NORMAL: 6 - 11 microns$^3$

## poisoning

These are substances which can do damage and for which there are blood tests. Corrosives (acids and alkalis) are not included; their damage is immediate and requires emergency attention. Some of the substances list a "toxic rating" because exposure can be fatal: class 6 is the most toxic, class 1 the least.

**acetaminophen**: pain medication, class 4

sources: over-the-counter drugs

symptoms: nausea, vomiting, abdominal pain, lethargy (after 24-36 hours), jaundice (after 48 hours); continued high doses will lead to liver damage. Notice that the symptoms appear long after its peak in the blood.

blood level: below 120 mcg/ml 4 hours after ingestion, toxicity is over 150 mcg/ml

**alcohol**: *ethyl alcohol*, class 2; see **alcohol**, page 15

sources: alcoholic beverages (beer, wine, etc.)

symptoms: slurred speech, slowed reflexes, depressed central nervous system function (consequently brain damage can occur with chronic abuse). Women who are able to conceive should be aware that alcohol can easily reach a developing fetus and do much damage before the woman even knows she is pregnant.

blood level: below 0.5 or 50 mg/dl in nonpregnant persons. No alcohol should be present during pregnancy.

**aluminum**: metallic element **Al**

sources: taken in from dialysis, antacids, most dentures, leaching from aluminum pots and pans, inhaled as bauxite fumes; external use: antiperspirant, astringent

**poisoning** (cont.)

symptoms: GI distress, if in blood can cause brain damage, accumulates in bone and hair, implicated in kidney failure and Alzheimer's

blood level: we can tolerate 3-10 mcg/l, patients on dialysis will usually have levels over 40 mcg/l

**antifreeze**: *ethylene glycol*, class 3

sources: automobile radiator additive

symptoms: slurred speech, slowed reflexes, much like alcohol intoxication; vomiting, seizures, coma. There can be kidney failure within 24-36 hours. Antifreeze containing *methanol* can cause blindness.

blood levels: none should be in the blood

**antimony**: metallic element **Sb**, class 6

sources: leaching of *antimony oxide* from enamelware by acid (e.g., acidic fruit juices), tartar emetic used to induce vomiting and to treat worms, fungi; industrial exposure (as a metal alloy, pigment in paint, fire-retardant, textile dye fixative) is not usually associated with poisoning

symptoms: like those of arsenic (interferes with cellular metabolism)

blood levels: below 1.0 mcg/l

**arsenic**: metallic element **As**, class 5

sources: most toxic are the inorganic forms ($AS^{3+}$ and $AS^{5+}$) primarily from pesticides (insect, rodent) and herbicides (weed killers), also metal adhesives, some chemotherapy drugs, some paints, wallpaper and ceramics, released into the atmosphere as a by-product of smelting. The organic forms found in food (shellfish) are nontoxic.

<u>symptoms</u>: abdominal pain from 2-12 hours after ingestion; muscle pain, difficulty urinating; chronic ingestion of low doses will lead to nervous system symptoms such as burning pains in the hands and feet

<u>blood levels</u>: below 3 mcg/dl; it will be in the blood less than 4 hours and will then accumulate in body tissue

**aspirin**: pain medication, class 4

<u>sources</u>: over-the-counter drugs, teething gel for infants

<u>symptoms</u>: abdominal pain, vomiting, dizziness, lethargy, ringing in the ears, hearing loss, fever, dehydration, restlessness, convulsions, coma. Chronic use can lead to bleeding and liver damage.

<u>blood level</u>: 2-20 mg/dl 2 hours after ingestion, toxicity is over 50 mg/dl. Toxicity in children can occur at much lower levels, particularly those with Reye's syndrome.

**asthma medication**: *bronchodilators*, class 4

<u>sources</u>: prescription and over-the-counter medication for asthma, bronchitis and emphysema. Coffee, tea and chocolate will increase blood levels, as will blood pressure reducing drugs, epinephrine (a hormone) and lithium (medication for manic-depression bipolar disorder), changes in blood pressure, flushing, sweating, convulsions, hallucinations, fever, chills, vomiting, clammy skin, stroke

<u>symptoms</u>: pounding heartbeat, dizziness, nervousness, bad taste in the mouth, dry mouth, headache, insomnia, anxiety,

<u>blood level</u>: *theophylline* 10-20 mcg/ml 2-3 hours after ingestion, toxicity is over 20 mcg/ml

### poisoning (cont.)

**barbiturates**: hypnotic, sedative or anesthetic, class 5
sources: prescription and over-the-counter drugs
symptoms: dizziness, headache, confusion, irregular heartbeat, low blood pressure, coma. Effects are made more severe with alcohol and other central nervous system depressants.
blood level: *phenobarbital* 10-40 mcg/ml, stays in system 8-16 hours, toxicity is over 70 mcg/ml; this is just one example.

**barium**: metallic element **Ba**
sources: insecticides (rat poison), fireworks, hair removers (*depilatories*), glass manufacturing, textile dying, food contamination
symptoms: muscle twitching, rigidity or weakness, heartbeat irregularities, anemia
blood levels: soon after ingestion of water-soluble barium salts

**bromide**: sedative
sources: some over-the-counter preparations (e.g., *Bromo-Seltzer*), well water, manufacture of photographic equipment/ paper
symptoms: skin rash, nausea, vomiting, GI irritation, weakness, constipation, central nervous system depression, mental deterioration (confusion, hallucinations, psychosis), anorexia, stupor, coma
blood levels: 1,000-2,000 µg/ml; toxicity greater than 3,000 µg/ml

**cadmium**: metallic element **Cd**, class 5
sources: by-product of zinc, lead, copper, arsenic mining and purification; widely used in manufacturing (especially of batteries and dental supplies), photography, printing, paints/

dyes, most food, plant oils and fats, alcohol, fish, poultry (zinc can neutralize some of the effects), preparation of food in vessels plated with cadmium (e.g., some cans), smoking. A blood test can confirm your exposure.

symptoms dermatitis with ulcers, drooling, nausea, vomiting, back and leg pain, difficulty breathing occurring within 15 minutes of ingestion and subsiding after 24 hours.

Inhalation of dust or vapor produces inflammation of the lungs. Chronic poisoning can cause loss of the sense of smell, coughing, difficulty breathing, Its presence is associated with cancer (lung, prostate), kidney dysfunction, diminished respiration, chronic lung disease, liver injury.

blood levels: below 10 ng/ml; with exposure, up to 40 ng/ml; toxicity seen at 50 ng/ml.

**caffeine**: stimulant, class 3

sources: kola nuts, cocoa beans, tea leaves, coffee beans; coffee, chocolate, medications, over-the-counter stimulants (e.g., *No-Doz*), cold preparations, pain medications

symptoms: headache, indigestion, insomnia, restlessness, nervousness, confusion, tremors, constipation, fever, irregular or rapid heartbeat, seizures; seems to exaggerate symptoms of schizophrenia and manic-depression

blood level: 5-20 µg/ml, toxicity over 30 µg/ml

**calcium**, metallic element **Ca**, see page 41; calcium poisoning is rare given the difficulty of absorbing it into the bloodstream; however environmental exposure to lungs, stomach and skin can do some damage

sources: *calcium carbonate* (chalk, a component in some toothpastes/powders and medicine, limestone), *calcium chloride* (drying agent, refrigerant, preservative, swimming pool additive, used on the road to control dust/ice), *calcium sulfate* ("plaster of Paris") symptoms: constipation, skin rash/burn, damage to mucous membranes, coughing

blood level would not be ordered, necessarily, to determine toxicity; a urine test would be more informative

**cantharide:** skin irritant from dried Spanish fly (also known as "blister bug"), class 6

sources: internal use as a diuretic and aphrodisiac

symptoms: burning in throat, GI pain; kidneys can fail

blood level: there should be none

**carbon monoxide, CO,** *carboxyhemoglobin,* gas, class 5, see p. 41

sources: smoking, automobile exhaust, fireplaces, barbecues and wood/coal stoves, charcoal briquettes, gas ranges, hot water heaters, dryers, kerosene heaters, oil burners

symptoms: similar to food poisoning: headache, dizziness, drowsiness, weakness, nausea, vomiting, rapid breathing, red skin, clumsiness, dim vision; can impair growth of a fetus; heart patients will be susceptible to heart attacks

blood level: 0%-3% for nonsmokers

**cardiac glycosides:** digitalis (class 4), **digitoxin** (class 5), **digoxin** (class 6)

sources: heart medication

symptoms: nausea, vomiting, diarrhea, blurred vision, disturbed heartbeat

blood level: digitoxin: 10-30 mcg/l; digoxin: 0.5-2.0 mcg/l

**chlorinated pesticides:** classes 5 and 6, (also referred to as chlorinated hydrocarbon pesticides) includes aldrin, dieldrin, endrin and endosulfan (very toxic), chlordane, DDT, heptachlor, kepone, lindane, mirex and toxaphene (moderately toxic), ethylan or perthane, hexachlorobenzene and methoxychlor (slightly toxic), chloroform, vinyl chloride and carbon tetrachloride (implicated as causing cancer); have been largely replaced by **organophosphates**

sources: agriculture (crop dusting), malaria control; usually ingested through the skin

symptoms: nausea, vomiting soon after exposure, interferes with transmission of nerve impulses ( especially in the brain) leading to confusion, behavior changes, involuntary movements, depressed respiration, tremors, seizures. coma; may cause kidney damage, cancer

blood level: none. Most labs will offer a screening test which will include some or most of the above.

**chlorinated phenols**: see **fungicides** and **PCP** below. Some labs group these substances together in a screening panel.

**chromium**: metallic element **Cr**, essential nutrient, required for the maintenance of normal glucose (appears to enhance the effects of insulin in glucose utilization) and aids the transport of amino acids to the liver and heart cells. (Chromium and nicotinic acid make up a substance called the *glucose tolerance factor*.)

sources: dietary: meats, brewer's yeast, whole grain cereals; industrial: (inhalation of chromium dust) in tanning, electroplating, steelmaking (soluble compounds are what cause problems)

symptoms: dermatitis, liver/kidney impairment, central nervous system damage, damage of nasal passage, bronchial asthma.. Low levels may diminish protein synthesis because of decreased utilization of amino acids.

blood level: 0.05-0.15 ng/ml. High levels normal at birth but decrease with age.

**cigarette smoke**, see **tobacco** below

**copper**: metallic element **Cu** and essential nutrient; usually detected with a urine test but is present in blood bound to a protein (*ceruloplasmin*, an alpha$_2$-globulin that binds about 95% of serum copper -- almost no copper exists in a free state in the blood) and is required for synthesis of hemoglobin;

**poisoning** (cont.)

sources: found in liver, oysters, beans, peas, avocado, whole grains (adult daily requirement 2 mg/day).

symptoms: nausea, vomiting, burning sensation in esophagus and stomach, diarrhea. Excreted in feces; small amount in urine. When toxicity is suspected, a urine test will be given rather than the blood test. Copper poisoning is possible: gradual accumulation, food contamination from utensils or copper salts.

blood tests:
    70 - 155 mcg/dl for serum copper
    20 - 45 mg/dl for ceruloplasmin or
    35 - 65 IU/dl: range is slightly higher from 6 months to age 12, lower in infants younger than 6 months;

High levels may indicate liver disease, anemia, heart attack, infection, liver disease, leukemia; false high may result from taking birth control pills, estrogens. Pregnancy will also elevate levels

**cyanide**, gas or salts, class 6

sources: fumigants, insecticides, rat poisons, metal polish, electroplating solutions; has been used in gas chambers; also in apple seeds, *Prunus* species pits (apricot, cherry, choke cherry, peach, plum and sloe), cassava beans, bitter almonds all of which will only release the cyanide if the outer shell is broken

symptoms: are rapid pulse, flushing, headache, dizziness, respiratory depression, loss of consciousness, convulsions; in its ionized state binds to hemoglobin and strangles the red blood cell. 80% of cyanide is converted to *thiocyanate* so you might want to test for that as well, particularly in patients being treated with sodium nitroprusside

blood level: less than 0.1 mg/l

blood level: less than 0.1 mg/l

**defoliant**: (paraquat), class 6, may be included in a "chlorinated phenols" screening panel

**fluoride**: *fluorine* is a toxic, gaseous element **F** that is combined with other elements to be useful, class 4

> sources: ant/roach/lice poisons, glass-making, "stannous fluoride" (topical application to protect teeth), dust from manufacturing. If you are at risk, a urine test taken before exposure and then after exposure will be used instead of a blood test. When combined with sodium, it can be ingested as supplements (as well as in treated water) and may be prescribed to increase bone density and calcification.
>
> symptoms: pain, salivation, nausea, vomiting, diarrhea, paralysis of the lung, heart failure; chronically high concentrations in water can mottle teeth, affect the bones and sometimes damage nerves/brain
>
> blood level: the test only detects fluoride at 0.1 mg/l. However, serum levels can reach 0.44 mg/l following a dose of 33-220 mg sodium fluoride (toxic: over 2.6 mg/l)

**food poisoning**:

> sources: from bacteria, viruses, protozoa, fungi on food or in the water used to prepare the food; from toxins in the food (mushrooms, green skin on potatoes) or sprayed on during growing.
>
> symptoms: onset varies: chemical poisoning may start in 30 minutes, 1-12 hours for bacteria, 12-48 hours for viruses and *salmonella*; nausea, vomiting, diarrhea, stomach pain except for *botulism* which usually only affects the nervous system
>
> blood level: it is preferable to keep a sample of the suspected food and have it tested. If you are tested, most common sources of food poisoning can be identified with an antibody blood test (page 27).

**poisoning** (cont.)

**fungicides**: mercury and copper compounds, pentachlorophenol, dithiocarbamates, tetramethylthiuram, disulfide, hexachlorobenzene, iodine, class 5, may be included in a "chlorinated phenols" screening panel

**general volatile** screening test: your lab will be able to tell you the substances sought; one panel includes *acetone, ethyl alcohol, isopropyl alcohol* and *methyl alcohol*, none of which are normally in the blood.

**gold**: metallic element **Au**
> sources: arthritis medication as gold salts
> symptoms: skin rash, bone marrow depression, jaundice, GI bleeding, headache, vomiting
> blood level: 0-1 µg/ml, toxic over 5 µg/ml

**heavy metals** evaluation: can include any of the *metallic elements*; one common panel tests for arsenic, **lead** and mercury.

**insecticides**, see *organophosphates* below

**iodine**: trace element **I**, class 5
> sources: medication (antiseptic, cough remedy), dyes, germicides, medicinal soaps, water treatment, photographic film, contrast media for X rays and fluroscopy
> symptoms: pimply rash, hives, asthma; it is a central nervous system depressant but is not easily absorbed: vomiting, diarrhea, abdominal pain, thirst, fever; food in the stomach neutralizes any toxic form into *iodide* which is harmless
> blood level: below 1.0 mcg/ml

**iron**: metallic element **Fe**, essential nutrient, see page 107
> sources: vitamin supplements, red meat (particularly liver), some enriched foods (e.g., cereal)
> symptoms: lethargy, vomiting, fast/weak pulse, low blood pressure, shock, pale skin
> blood level: 25-200 mcg/dl

**lead**: metallic element **Pb**, class 5, see page 114
**lithium**: metallic element **Li**, class 5
> sources: medication (manic-depression, alcoholism, leukemia)
> symptoms: tremors, twitching, apathy, difficulty speaking, anorexia, hair loss, dry mouth, blurred vision, confusion, coma
> blood level: 0.5-1.3 mEq/l

**magnesium**, metallic element **Mg**, essential nutrient, see page 123.
> sources: food, vitamin supplements, antacids, laxatives; industrial exposure in structural alloys, fireworks, flash photography, incendiary bombs
> symptoms: lethargy, red face, sweating, low blood pressure, slow/weak pulse, slow reflexes, muscle weakness, shallow breathing
> blood level: 1.2-3.0 mg/dl

**manganese**, metallic element **Mn**, trace mineral, see page 124.
> sources: mining, metalworking, foundry work, welding, exposure to paint, fertilizer, the manufacturing of drugs/ glass/steel/dry-cell batteries, food, vitamin supplements, contaminated water
> symptoms: usually from inhalation rather than ingestion, central nervous systems disorders (Parkinson's disease, psychiatric disorders, brain damage), impaired movement, edema (retaining water), liver disease, lung infection
> blood level: 0.04 - 1.4 mcg/dl

**mercury** metallic element **Hg**
> sources: can be absorbed through the skin and mucous membranes as well as eaten in contaminated food (usually fish). Some professions are susceptible: dental assistants, mirror/thermometer manufacturers, use/manufacture of insecticides

**poisoning** (cont.)

symptoms: vomiting, diarrhea, kidney failure, weakness, brain damage, loss of balance, mental illness, muscle pain. It can't be eliminated from the body, so will accumulate in the kidneys.

blood level: 0 - 1 or 2 mcg/dl

**minerals** (trace elements): Like vitamins, some minerals need to be gotten from food in order for the body to function properly (calcium, magnesium, manganese, phosphorus, zinc). However, some (e.g., lead, mercury) do nothing for the body but will probably be found in the body and can be measured.

**narcotics**: depressants, classes 5 and 6: codeine, heroin, morphine, opium, paragoric

sources: prescription drugs, "street" drugs

symptoms: initial stimulation, then drowsiness, headache, slow and shallow breathing, coma

blood level: none

**nerve gas**, see **organophosphates** below

**nickel**: metallic element **Ni**, can be toxic when inhaled but is usually measured with a urine test.

sources: innumerable household products (doorknobs, zippers, razors, etc.), astringents, dyes (including hair dyes), textile printing, coatings, ceramics

symptoms: skin rash, nausea, vomiting, diarrhea, central nervous system damage, lung disease, kidney damage

blood level: 1-8 mcg/l

**nicotine**: plant alkaloid, class 6, see also **tobacco** below

sources: insecticides, tobacco products, stop-smoking products

symptoms: first stimulates then depresses the central nervous system (brain and spinal cord); can influence involuntary body functions: slow heart rate, nausea, vomiting in non-habitual

users but in habitual users nearly the opposite effect: raising blood pressure, improving concentration, eliminating fatigue
blood level: none; it may be worthwhile to ask for a test if you are concerned about secondary smoke; your lab might test directly for nicotine or might measure the levels of either *cotinine* or *polyaromatic hydrocarbons*

**organophosphates**: organic pesticides, all classes of toxicity
sources: malathion, carbamates, diazanon, TEPP (tetra-ethylpyrophosphate), parathion, flea and tick collars, muscle relaxants, nerve gas, manufacture of lubricants, fire retardants, and pesticides (ingestion can be absorption through the skin as well as inhalation and swallowing)
symptoms: headache, cramps, vomiting, diarrhea, dizziness, weakness, sweating, drooling, skin and kidney disease, psychosis. Interferes with the enzyme *cholinesterase* which helps to regulate both the central nervous system and the parasympathetic nervous system (look for pinpoint-sized pupils and muscle twitching).
blood level: *cholinesterase*: 0.5 or above pH units/hour (serum), 0.7 or above pH units/hour (red blood cells); the lower the value, the greater the likelihood of phosphate poisoning. *Acetylcholinesterase* is an enzyme which lets a muscle fiber relax and recover; it is present in nerve tissue, spleen and brain; blood levels range from 11,000-15,000 IU/l; the higher the level, the more likely to be insecticide poisoning. The enzyme *pseudocholinesterase* performs a similar function, is produced in the liver and found in the pancreas, intestine, heart and brain, and should be present in the blood at levels from 8 - 18 IU/ml; the lower the level, the more likely to be insecticide poisoning (or an inherited deficiency).

**poisoning** (cont.)

**oxalates**: *oxalic acid* and its salts, class 4
<u>sources</u>: car radiator cleaners, laundry bleach, fabric manufacture/cleaning, house plants (*dieffenbachia, philodendron*)
<u>symptoms</u>: skin/mucous membrane irritation, swelling of throat, kidney damage
<u>blood level</u>: below 27 mmol/l; usually measured with a urine test
**PCBs**: *polychlorinated biphenyls*, 209 compounds; banned in 1976 but is long-lived and has gotten into our food chain.
<u>sources</u>: transformers, capacitors, printing ink, paints, dusting agents, pesticides, occupational exposure, contaminated fish; major source of exposure today includes spills or landfill leaching of waste oils from industrial sources.
<u>symptoms</u>: (from inhalation, ingestion, absorption), skin disease/discoloration, swelling, nausea, vomiting, abdominal pain, liver damage, blindness; cannot be excreted from the body
<u>blood level</u>: below 16 mg/ml, detectable in about ½ of adult US population. Accumulates in fatty tissue at concentrations approximately 190 times the blood level; dermatologic symptoms occur at 44 ng/ml; neurological effects at 75 ng/ml including suppression of the immune system
**PCP**: *phencyclidine* also known as "angel dust", class 6, may be included in a "chlorinated phenols" screening panel
<u>sources</u>: anesthesia, sedative, veterinary drugs
<u>symptoms</u>: lethargy, euphoria, hallucinations, agitation, violent behavior, fever, high blood pressure, rigidity, rapid heartbeat, convulsions, kidney failure, brain damage, coma
<u>blood level</u>: none should be in your body

**pesticides**: The suffix "-cide" identifies a killing agent: insecticide kills insects, algaecide kills algae, fungicide kills fungi, herbicide kills plants, rodenticide kills rodents, etc. See also arsenic, chlorinated pesticides, cyanide, fluoride, fungicides, mercury, nicotine, organophosphates, PCBs.

**phosphorus**: non-metallic element **P** and essential nutrient, in white/yellow (which ignites on contact with moist air or water), red (made from white when exposed to heat or sunlight, nontoxic) and black forms (made from white under high pressure, nontoxic), class 6

> sources: organophosphates (malathion), rat poison, manufacture of fertilizer, matches and fireworks
>
> symptoms: stomach pain/acidity, nausea, vomiting, diarrhea, then a period of no symptoms during which liver, heart, kidney and nervous system are damaged, then more intense symptoms recur after 3 days; can burn skin; inhalation can cause eye infection, nausea, vomiting, fatigue, cough, jaundice, tremors, numbness, low blood pressure, fluid in the lungs, heart irregularities, convulsions. Chronic poisoning is characterized by a "phossy jaw," aching and swelling of the jaw followed by deterioration of the jawbone plus weakness, weight loss, anemia and spontaneous fractures
>
> blood level: 2.3 - 4.7 mg/dl of "inorganic phosphorus"

**potassium**: metallic element **K** and essential nutrient, classes 4 and 5, see page 159.

> sources: food (dates, apricots, bananas, oranges, tomatoes, iodized table salt, cream of tartar), antiseptic/astringent (in toothpaste, mouthwash, gargles), drugs, disinfectant, wood cleaners, ink-stain and paint removers, printing ink, black dye, photography, explosives, fireworks, matches, manufacturing (of soap, glass, pottery, adhesives), fertilizer, plant food, salt substitute, buffer solution, fur processing, insecticides

**poisoning** (cont.)

symptoms: skin rash, disorientation, weakness, low blood pressure, burning in throat, nausea, vomiting, difficulty swallowing or swollen throat, dry mouth, eventual kidney damage

blood level: 3.5 - 5.5 mEq/l

**selenium**: metallic element and essential nutrient **Se**

sources: soil, photoelectric cells, light meters, photocopying machines, electrical components, part of the red color in warning lights, traffic lights and brake lights; dietary sources are meat, fish (especially shellfish), dairy products

symptoms: pale skin, garlic breath, metallic taste in the mouth, stomach upset, nose irritation, eye infection, skin problems, drowsiness, tightness of the chest

blood level: 85-125 ng/ml

**silver**: metallic element **Ag**, class 5

sources: astringent to treat eye infection and burns

symptoms: burning in mouth, blackened skin/mucous membranes/throat, vomiting, diarrhea, collapse. Chronic exposure will turn the skin blue-black.

blood level: below 0.2 μg/ml

**sodium**: metallic element **Na** and essential nutrient (page 177), classes 3 and 4

sources: part of innumerable common compounds (from *sodium acetate* to *sodium xylenesulfonate*) so the first level of safety is not to ingest questionable substances. Nonfood: medicines (especially corticosteroids and blood pressure reducers), mouthwash, toothpaste; high sodium food: baking powder, baking soda, barbecue sauce, bouillon cubes, cake, carbonated beverages, chili sauce, condiments (ketchup, mustard, etc.), cookies, cooking wine, garlic salt, nondairy creamer, softened water, soy sauce.

symptoms: thirst, restlessness, dry/sticky mucous membranes, flushed skin, reduced urine output, diminished reflexes, labored breathing, high blood pressure, water retention; ingesting salt water has been known to bring on heart attack

blood level: 135 - 145 mEq/l

**thallium**: metallic element **Tl**, class 6

sources: rat poison, depilatories (chemical hair removers), inorganic chemical insecticides, flue dust, manufacture of glasses/photoelectric cells/costume jewelry/low temperature thermometers (easily absorbed by skin and GI tract), can affect developing fetus from maternal exposure

symptoms: hair loss, pain in hands/feet, fever, eye infection, stomach pain, nausea, bloody diarrhea, lethargy, tremors, convulsions, pneumonia, personality changes, anxiety, depression, psychotic behavior

blood level: below 10 ng/ml

**tobacco**: *Nicotiana* species of plant, class 4, see nicotine above.

sources: eating fresh leaves, enemas, chewing tobacco, cigarettes, cigars

symptoms: anxiety, irritability, confusion, halting speech, dizziness, sleepiness, nausea, vomiting, loss of appetite, ringing in ears, cough, irregular pulse

blood level: none

**vitamin A**: *retinol*, essential nutrient, see page 193.

sources: dietary supplements, acne treatment, polar bear liver (just in case you encounter it on an adventure)

symptoms: peeling skin, hair loss, irritability, anorexia, swollen legs/arms, bleeding lips, headache, craving for butter, changes in menstruation and skin pigmentation, liver and kidney damage

blood level: 30-95 mcg/dl

poisoning (cont.)

**vitamin C**: *ascorbic acid*, essential nutrient, see page 197.
sources: dietary supplements, citrus fruits, vegetables
symptoms: diarrhea, (converted to an oxalate, see page 153 above, in the body which can lead to kidney problems with chronic overexposure)
blood level: 0.2-2.0 mg/dl

**vitamin D**: essential nutrient, see page 197.
sources: dietary supplements, sunshine (which does not contribute to a buildup in the body)
symptoms: weakness, fatigue, loss of appetite, nausea, vomiting, yellowish deposits under fingernails/in the eyes/ over the skin, failure to grow (in children), calcium toxicity
blood level: 24-65 pg/ml

**vitamin E**: *tocopherol* compounds, essential nutrient, see page 199
sources: dietary supplements, plant oils, leaves of green vegetables
symptoms: swollen lips, headache, dizziness, fatigue, muscle weakness, high blood pressure, allergies, GI distress, nausea, disruption of iron metabolism
blood level: 5-20 mcg/ml

**vitamin K**: *naphthoquinone* compounds and essential nutrient, see page 200.
sources: dietary supplements, plant leaves
symptoms: problems with overclotting of the blood (e.g., phlebitis)
blood level: 0.09 - 2.2 ng/ml

**zinc**: metallic element **Zn** and essential nutrient, class 5, see page 211.
sources: water, food (meat, seafood, dairy products, whole grains, nuts, legumes), dietary supplements, fumes (metal work and manufacturing, paint and rubber manufacturing), drinking from galvanized cans

<u>symptoms</u>: irritate the skin as well as the respiratory and GI tracts; oral poisoning (uncommon) is caused by and produces fever and GI distress, metallic taste in mouth, dry throat, cough, chest pain

<u>blood level</u>: 60-150 mcg/dl

## potassium
### (serum potassium, $K^+$)

DESCRIPTION: A positively charged electrolyte found in large amounts in all cells; regulates the enzymes responsible for metabolizing starches and sugars. Can also affect the regularity of the heartbeat.

Obtained from the diet (from beef, chicken, scallops and veal; artichokes, asparagus, beans, broccoli, carrots, mushrooms, potatoes, spinach, squash, tomatoes and tomato juice; apricots, apricot nectar, bananas, cantaloupe, figs, grapefruit juice, orange juice, peaches, pears, pineapple juice and prune juice); excreted by the kidneys.

TEST TYPE: venous blood, chemistry

TEST OF: kidney, adrenal glands

TEST FOR: level in blood

HOW OFTEN: with symptoms; during use of digitalis (heart medication)

NORMAL: 3.5 - 5.5 mEq/l. *Consult range given by your lab.*

HIGH: Addison's disease, adrenal gland deficiency, breathing restriction, burns, cell damage, crushing injuries, diabetic complications, heart attack, kidney failure, too much potassium (see page 154)

FALSE HIGH: environment: tobacco

LOW: adrenal gland overactivity, Cushing's syndrome

FALSE LOW:

- <u>drugs</u>: blood pressure reducers, diuretics (acetazolamide), hormones (ACTH, cortisone), TB medication (para-aminosalicylic acid)
- <u>environment</u>: diarrhea, loss of body fluids, eating too much licorice
- <u>medical</u>: improper administration of glucose or insulin

## pregnancy

No woman has to be told her entire body chemistry changes with pregnancy. Here is a list of how blood tests will be affected.

| Values Will Decrease | Values Will Increase |
|---|---|
| **albumin** | alkaline **phos**phatase |
| **bicarbonate** | **chloride** |
| **calcium** | **cholesterol** |
| **creatinine** | **CPK** (late pregnancy) |
| hematocrit (**HCT**) | **glucose** |
| hemoglobin (**Hgb**) | **LD** |
| pCO$_2$ (**CO$_2$**) | leukocytes (**WBC**) |
| **phosphorus** | **sedi**mentation **rate** |
| SGOT (**AST**) | |
| **sodium** | |
| urea nitrogen (**BUN**) | |

COMMENTS: The **hCG** test, page 86, will tell you if you are pregnant. To check the health of the developing fetus, see **AFP** (page 9), **fetal monitoring** (page 72) and **TORCH** (page 187) tests.

**prenatal** tests, see **fetal monitoring**, page 72.

## pro time
### (prothrombin time, PT)

OTHER NAMES: Factor II

DESCRIPTION: There are twelve "factors" involved in making a blood clot, the body's instant bandage. Prothrombin is a protein which is one of the factors.

*Fibrin* is a type of protein that's essential to the clotting of blood (see page 73). The pro time test measures how long it takes for a fibrin clot to form in a specially treated blood sample.

TEST TYPE:      venous blood, rheology

TEST OF:      coagulation

TEST FOR:      clotting time, by calculation

HOW OFTEN:      as needed for drug therapy; prior to surgery

NORMAL:

- 11.0 - 18.0 sec or 100% of control time in adults
- 70% - 100% of control time in children. *Consult the range given on your lab sheet.*

SLOW:      bile duct obstruction, liver disease, bleeding problems

FALSE SLOW:

- <u>drugs</u>: antibiotics, anticoagulant (alone or with alcohol, analgesics, anti-inflammatory medication, aspirin, epilepsy medication, heartbeat regulators, thyroid hormones, malaria medication, vitamin A), barbiturates, pain relievers, sedatives, TB

medication
- nutrition: vitamin K deficiency
- environment: use of mineral oil

COMMENTS: This is not the same test as the *thrombin clotting time* test, not included in this volume.

### protein
#### (total serum protein)

DESCRIPTION: ***Albumin, globulin*** and *fibrinogen* are the protein components of blood. Only the first two are included in the protein total. (See COMMENTS, next page.) Their ratio -- **a/g ratio** -- also aids in diagnosis.

Proteins are not stored in the body but are broken down into amino acids (and **ammonia**, then into *urea* which is how the body disposes of nitrogen, see **BUN**). Since we have no reservoir of protein in the body, good nutrition must supply this in our diet.

TEST TYPE: venous blood, chemistry

TEST OF: liver

TEST FOR: level in blood by calculation (sum of albumin and globulin levels)

HOW OFTEN: regular physical exam

NORMAL:
- 6.0 - 8.0 gm/dl
- levels will be lower in infants. *Consult ranges given by your lab.*

**protein** (cont.)

**a/g ratio**: 1.5 - 2.5/l (notice that albumin levels will be roughly twice those of globulin

HIGH:          arthritis, cancer, chronic inflammatory disease (e.g., rheumatoid arthritis), dehydration (from vomiting, diarrhea), diabetic acidosis, infection. If the proportion of globulin increases, this may indicate that the walls of the red blood cells are weakening (allowing albumin to leak out).

LOW:          burns, diabetes, heart failure, hemorrhage, Hodgkin's disease, intestinal malabsorption, kidney disease, liver dysfunction, malnutrition, poisoning (benzene, carbon tetrachloride), overactive thyroid, toxemia (of pregnancy)

FALSE LOW:
- drugs: birth control pills, laxatives
- environment: pregnancy, sustained reclining position (as in prolonged illness or bed rest), surgery, tourniquet left on too long prior to test

COMMENTS: *Fibrinogen* is eliminated from the blood sample (in order to measure albumin and globulin) by allowing a clot to form in the sample and then using the remaining fluid -- now properly *serum* -- to measure the two remaining proteins.

## PSA
**(prostate-specific antigen)**

DESCRIPTION: An *antigen* is any substance that evokes a response from the immune system (this can include dissolved toxins, bacteria, etc.). In general, some kinds of tumor cells will release unique substances in the blood. If we can identify such a substance, we can infer the presence of a tumor and seek to find it in the body's tissue. PSA is such a **tumor marker.**

TEST TYPE:     venous blood, chemistry

TEST OF:       prostate gland

TEST FOR:      level in blood

HOW OFTEN:     abnormality of prostate; normal exam as men age

NORMAL:        **men**
- below 2 ng/ml African Americans in their 40's*
  below 2.5 ng/ml others in their 40's*
- below 4 ng/ml African Americans in their 50's,60's
  below 3.5 ng/ml others in their 50's
  below 4.5 ng/ml others in their 60's
- below 5.5 ng/ml African Americans in their 70's
  below 6.5 ng/ml others in their 70's
  *Consult ranges given by your lab.*

HIGH:          prostate cancer, prostate disease

FALSE HIGH:    prostate massage or surgery

COMMENTS:  A more specialized test measures *free PSA*, which distinguishes cancer from benign conditions.

*There is active disagreement about whether screening should begin below age 50.

## PTT
### (partial thromboplastin time)

OTHER NAMES: activated partial thromboplastin time (APTT)

DESCRIPTION: *Thromboplastin* is one of the **clotting factors** and is used in testing to measure how long it takes the blood to form a clot. It is made from tissue. *Partial thromboplastin* is made from platelets and clots more slowly. Often ordered with the **pro time** test (page 161) to aid in diagnosis.

TEST TYPE: venous blood, rheology

TEST OF: blood coagulation

TEST FOR: clotting factors

HOW OFTEN: to monitor heparin drug therapy; abnormal bleeding; prior to surgery; at birth to check for clotting factor deficiencies

NORMAL: 25 - 50 seconds (along with a time for a control sample). *Consult the range given on your lab sheet.*

SLOW: bile duct obstruction, liver disease, deficiency of clotting factors

FALSE SLOW: drugs: heparin or any other circulating anti-coagulant

## RBC
### (red blood cell count)

DESCRIPTION: Number of circulating red blood cells in a one $mm^3$ (cubic millimeter) sample. Follow the ranges given on your lab sheet as many variables affect the sample: age, gender, handling, geographic location (altitude).

TEST TYPE: venous blood, capillary blood (from newborns), hematology, CBC

TEST OF: blood

TEST FOR: concentration of red blood cells

HOW OFTEN: regular physical exam

NORMAL:
- 4.7 - 6.1 million/$mm^3$ in men
- 4.2 - 5.4 million/$mm^3$ in women
- 3.8 - 5.5 million/$mm^3$ in children
- 4.8 - 7.1 million/$mm^3$ in newborns. *Consult ranges given by your lab.*

HIGH: blood or bone marrow disease, dehydration, heart disease

FALSE HIGH: environment: high altitude

LOW: anemia, bone marrow failure, chronic illness, excessive bleeding, fluid overload, iron deficiency, organ failure, vitamin $B_{12}$ deficiency

**RBC** (cont.)

FALSE LOW:     drugs: chemotherapy, malaria medication

## RBC indices
**(red blood cell indices: MCV, MCH, MCHC)**

OTHER NAMES: RBC indexes, erythrocyte indices

DESCRIPTION: Uses the results of the **RBC**, hematocrit (**HCT**), and hemoglobin (**Hgb**) tests to calculate a quantitative profile of the red blood cells, the make-up of the actual cell mass. Helps to distinguish types of anemia.

TEST TYPE:     venous blood, hematology, CBC

TEST OF:       blood

TEST FOR:      volume

HOW OFTEN:     with symptoms of anemia

**Mean corpuscular volume** (MCV) is the measure of the average volume of a single red blood cell and is calculated as the ratio of hematocrit to the RBC count. This will indicate whether the cells are of normal size, "normocytic." If they are too small, your lab sheet will refer to them as "microcytic," too large as "macrocytic." High white blood cell count (WBC) will invalidate this measure.

NORMAL:
- 80 - 96 microns$^3$ in adults and children
- 96 - 108 microns$^3$ in newborns.

HIGH:                    alcoholism, anemia (from deficiency of folic acid/vitamin $B_{12}$)

LOW:                     iron-deficiency anemia, hemoglobin disorder (e.g., thalassemia)

**Mean corpuscular hemoglobin** (MCH) is the average weight of hemoglobin in an average red blood cell (the hemoglobin to RBC ratio). High white blood cell count (WBC) and false high hemoglobin will invalidate this measure.

NORMAL:

- 23 - 31 pg in adults and children
- 32 - 34 pg in newborns. *Consult ranges given by your lab.*

**Mean corpuscular hemoglobin concentration** (MCHC) is the amount of hemoglobin in an average red blood cell (the ratio of hemoglobin to hematocrit). Helps to distinguish normally colored RBCs ("normochromic") from paler cells ("hypochromic"). False high hemoglobin will invalidate this measure.

NORMAL:

- 32 - 36 g/dl or
  32% - 36% in adults and children
- 32 - 33 g/dl or
  32% - 33% in newborns. *Consult ranges given by your lab.*

LOW:                     iron-deficiency anemia, hemoglobin disorder (e.g., thalassemia)

## retic count
### (reticulocyte count)

DESCRIPTION: *Reticulocytes* are immature red blood cells.

TEST TYPE:     capillary or venous blood, hematology

TEST OF:     bone marrow function

TEST FOR:     bone marrow activity

HOW OFTEN:     to evaluate treatment of anemia

NORMAL:

- 0.5 - 2% in adults (This means there are about 0.1-1.5 reticulocytes per 100 red blood cells.)
- 0.5 - 3.1% in infants
- 2.5 - 6.5% in newborns. *Consult ranges given by your lab*

HIGH:     overproduction of RBC's

FALSE HIGH:     <u>drugs</u>: antibiotics (sulfonamides), antimalarials, fever reducers, iron, parasite treatment (furazolidone), Parkinson's medication (L-dopa)

LOW:     anemia (from deficiency of folic acid or vitamin $B_{12}$)

FALSE LOW:     <u>drugs</u>: antibiotics (chloramphenicol, dactinomycin, sulfonamides), chemotherapy (methotrexate) or any drug affecting the bone marrow (azathioprine)

# RF

## (rheumatoid factor)

OTHER NAMES: RA, RAF, rheumatoid arthritis factor

DESCRIPTION: Antibody to one of the body's white blood cells (specifically, a B lymphocyte or **immunoglobulin**). This is an instance of *autoimmunity*, "immunity to one's own immune system."

TEST TYPE: venous blood, serology

TEST OF: immune system

TEST FOR: presence of antibody

HOW OFTEN: with symptoms of arthritis

NORMAL: negative (no presence of antibody, or a titer of less than 1:20, see **serology**, page 173). As the body ages, there may be low levels of antibodies without having rheumatoid arthritis.

FALSE NEGATIVE: some people can have rheumatoid arthritis without a positive RF titer; also it takes 6 months after the onset of disease for RF to become reactive.

POSITIVE: *Levels between 1:20 and 1:80*
heart disease, liver disease, lung disease, lupus, mononucleosis, scleroderma (hardening of the skin), syphilis, thyroid disease, tuberculosis, worms

**RF** (cont.)

*Levels over 1:80*
rheumatoid arthritis

FALSE POSITIVE: <u>medical</u>: blood with high lipid levels or blood
protein disorder

## Rh type

DESCRIPTION: Rh is a protein that appears on a red blood cell,
specifically the **$Rh_0(D)$ antigen**. When the protein is present, the
blood is said to be "Rh positive." Introducing Rh positive blood into
a person with no protein ("Rh negative") will cause an antibody
reaction to occur. If antibodies are already present, the reaction is
likely to be fatal.
    Your lab sheet may refer to "$D^u$ variants." If your classification is
"$Rh(D^u)$ positive" this means that the protein is very weakly expressed
and you can receive either Rh-positive or Rh-negative blood.

TEST TYPE:     capillary or venous blood, serology

TEST OF:       blood

TEST FOR:      subtype

HOW OFTEN:     at birth; prior to surgery or transfusion; onset of
               pregnancy

FALSE POSITIVE (for $D^u$ variant): <u>drugs</u>: antibiotics (cephalo-
                    sporins), blood pressure reducers (methyldopa),
                    Parkinson's medication (L-dopa)

## sed rate

### (sedimentation rate)

OTHER NAMES: erythrocyte sedimentation rate (ESR)

DESCRIPTION: Speed at which the red blood cells separate from plasma and settle. This test is often the earliest indication of disease although it can't tell you which disease. Settling time gradually increases with age (i.e., will tend toward slow values).

TEST TYPE:        venous blood, hematology

TEST OF:          immune system

TEST FOR:         rate of settling (to inform of condition of blood)

HOW OFTEN:        screening for infection, disease severity

NORMAL:
- 0 - 9 mm/hour in men
- 0 - 15 mm/hour in women
- 0 - 20 mm/hr in children. *Consult ranges given by your lab.*

Westergren method
- 0 - 15 mm/hour in men
  0 - 20 mm/hour over age 50
- 0 - 20 mm/hour in women
  0 - 30 mm/hour over age 50

FAST:             anemia, autoimmune disease (e.g., rheumatoid arthritis), cancer, heart attack, infection, inflammation, kidney disease, rheumatic fever,

**sed rate** (cont.)

thyroid disease, tuberculosis, tumor

FALSE FAST:      <u>environment</u>: pregnancy

SLOW:            sickle-cell anemia, liver disease

FALSE SLOW:      <u>environment</u>: sample allowed to stand too long

**selenium**
See **poisoning**, page 155.

**serology**

DESCRIPTION: Analyzes serum for **antibodies**, immune complexes, antigen-antibody reactions.

TEST TYPE:       venous blood

TEST OF:         indirectly: spleen, lymph nodes, bone marrow and thymus gland (where antibodies are made)

TEST FOR:        presence of antibodies in blood

HOW OFTEN:
- at birth (for blood group and Rh factor)
- prior to transfusion (*direct Coombs* and *indirect Coombs* tests)
- when pregnancy is possible
- outbreak of disease in your area or exposure to a known infection

COMMENTS: Your lab sheet may refer to "titers" or "neutralization tests." This is a specific type of test used in serology. A live virus is added to a blood sample. If antibodies are present, they will bind to the virus and keep it from infecting the body -- they neutralize the virus. To find out how much antibody is in the blood (the "level" so to speak), an *estimation* is made by diluting the blood. The lab will test for neutralization each time the blood is diluted. The highest dilution which neutralizes the virus is called an *antibody titer*.


**SGOT** (serum glutamic oxalacetic transaminase)
See **AST** (aspartate aminotransferase), page 31.

**SGPT** (serum glutamic pyruvic transaminase)
See **ALT** (alanine aminotransferase), page 21.

## sickle cell screening
### (hemoglobin S test)

DESCRIPTION: Hemoglobin S (often with hemoglobin C and sometimes A) can distort the shape of red blood cells, preventing normal flow of blood. This blood screen is meant to determine only the actual presence of "sickling hemoglobins."

However, it is common to request a prenatal diagnosis for high risk couples to detect genetic mutations in a fetus. In this case, amniotic fluid is tested along with the mother's blood. A family history is usually required.

TEST TYPE:      capillary blood, hematology

TEST OF:        red blood cells

TEST FOR:       shape and behavior or cells

HOW OFTEN:      at birth

NORMAL:         absence of sickle cells

COMMENTS: It is well known that persons of African descent are more likely to have cells that sickle. However, it is certainly not limited to this particular group. If your ancestors come from an area having malaria, your risk increases. Additionally, anyone could have an ancestor from an affected group without being aware of it.

Genetic testing is available to determine if you suffer from the anemia or are a carrier, or to determine the status of a fetus from carrier or afflicted parents.

**silver**
See **poisoning**, page 155.

# SMA
## (Sequential Multiple Analyzer)

DESCRIPTION: This is a machine that analyzes blood tests simultaneously and is one of the standard screening tests most frequently ordered. Which type of SMA will depend on which machine your lab uses. Examples are:

**SMA-12**: (In the Midwest, this is called the SMA 12/60.) albumin, alk phos, AST, bilirubin, BUN, calcium, cholesterol, glucose, in phos, LD, protein, uric acic

**SMA-23**: a/g ratio, albumin, alk phos, ALT, AST, bilibrubin, BUN, BUN/creat ratio, calcium, carbon dioxide, chloride, cholesterol, creatinine, globulin, glucose, in phos, iron total, LD, potassium, protein, sodium, triglycerides, uric acid

**SMAC**: a/g ratio, albumin, alk phos, ALT, anion gap, AST, bilirubin, BUN, BUN/creat ratio, calcium, carbon dioxide, chloride, cholesterol, cholesterol/HDL ratio, creatinine, ferritin, GGTP, globulin, glucose, HDL cholesterol, in phos, ionized calcium, LD, LDL cholesterol, LDL/HDL ratio, osmolality, phos, potassium, protein, sodium, triglycerides, uric acid

## sodium

### (serum sodium, Na$^+$)

DESCRIPTION: A positively charged **electrolyte** (page 63) essential for maintaining the proper balance of fluids in the body as well as helping nerve/muscle function, **pH, chloride** levels and **potassium** levels. Obtained mostly through salt in the diet.

TEST TYPE: venous blood, chemistry

TEST OF: kidney, adrenal glands, neuromuscular function

TEST FOR: level in blood

HOW OFTEN: regular physical exam; suspected electrolyte imbalance

NORMAL: 135 - 145 mEq/l. *Consult range given by your lab.*

HIGH: dehydration (from hyperventilation, vomiting, diarrhea), diabetes, heart failure, kidney disease, overdose (see page 155)

FALSE HIGH:
- <u>diet</u>: high salt intake, low fluid intake
- <u>drugs</u>: blood pressure medication, diuretics, steroids
- <u>environment</u>: burns, water loss (e.g., sweating)

LOW: adrenal overactivity, alkaline deficit, burns, poor kidney function (chronic)

FALSE LOW:
- <u>diet</u>: too little salt
- <u>drugs</u>: blood pressure reducers, diuretics, steroids

- environment: excessive fluid loss (vomiting, sweating, diarrhea)

COMMENTS: Because so much of our food is processed and loaded with sodium, we usually need to *reduce* dietary intake to not overload our system. Increasing intake of fresh food and being alert to the uses of sodium (in soda, nondairy substitutes, softened water, antacids for indigestion, aspirin, cough medicine, mouthwash, toothpaste as well as in processed food) will help to keep our sodium intake within reasonable limits.

**T-cell count**
See **WBC diff,** T-lymphocytes, page 208.

# $T_3$
## (serum triiodothyronine)

DESCRIPTION: $T_3$ is the most active of the thyroid hormones. The purpose of the thyroid gland is introduced on page 185. It is the hormones that carry out this purpose, primarily increasing the rate of body cell reactions.

In order to travel the bloodstream to get to the body's cells, they are usually attached to a protein (a *thyroid-binding protein*). The amount "taken up" by the protein is measured in the *$T_3$ uptake* test. When the hormones arrive at their destination, they are released. This means that some $T_3$ is "free" in the blood (*$FT_3$*) and can also be measured.

The **$T_3$** test indirectly measures the <u>total</u> level of triiodothyronine by adding the levels of bound $T_3$ and unbound $T_3$. In other words,

$$T_3 = FT_3 + T_3 \text{ uptake}$$

($T_3$ uptake is also used as a measure of thyroxine, **$T_4$**, page 181.) An *$rT_3$* test (*reverse $T_3$*) is used to tell if your symptoms aren't caused by the thyroid.

TEST TYPE:    venous blood, chemistry

TEST OF:    thyroid gland

TEST FOR:    level in blood

HOW OFTEN:    at birth; healthy women over 35 should be evaluated more regularly; with symptoms

NORMAL:    **$T_3$** 90 - 250 ng/dl
**$FT_3$** 0.2 - 0.6 ng/dl
**$T_3u$** 22% - 38% (is bound to protein)
**$rT_3$** 30 - 60 ng/dl. *Consult ranges given by your lab.*

HIGH:                     acute liver disease, overactive thyroid; if $T_4$ level is normal, suggests Graves' disease, tumors or swelling of the thyroid gland

FALSE HIGH:

- <u>drugs</u>: anticoagulants or blood thinners
- <u>environment</u>: cold weather, high altitude, pregnancy
- <u>medical</u>: hormone replacement therapy, tests using iodine (within six months)

LOW:                      excess sex hormones (androgens and estrogens), injury, kidney disease, liver disease, malnutrition, underactive thyroid

FALSE LOW:

- <u>drugs</u>: aspirin, birth control pills, epilepsy medication, steroids
- <u>environment</u>: aging, hot weather, surgery

COMMENTS: For the very curious among you, the subscripts in $T_3$ and $T_4$ are assigned following the rules of arithmetic which usually govern superscripts. $T_1$ (*monoiodotyrosine*) and $T_2$ (*diiodotyrosine*) are amino acids formed when iodine is added to the amino acid *tyrosine*. $T_3$ is formed by joining a molecule of $T_1$ with a molecule of $T_2$; $T_4$ is formed by joining two $T_2$ molecules. (And $T_7$ is formed by multiplying $T_4$ times $T_3u$, see COMMENTS in **$T_4$** test.)

# T₄
## (serum thyroxine)

DESCRIPTION: Another thyroid hormone, the levels of *free thyroxine* (FT₄) and *bound* (TBG) together account for the total thyroxine in the blood. **T₄** is converted to **T₃** mostly in the liver (only a small amount is made in the thyroid gland). TBG (*thyroxine-binding globulin*) carries <u>both</u> T₃ and T₄ through the blood.

When given to a newborn, the test is sometimes referred to as a screen for *congenital hypothyroidism*. Affecting more girls than boys, an absence (or very low levels) of T₄ can result in irreversible brain damage by age 3 months. Consequently, some states require the test at birth. If the levels are low, a complete thyroid function series will be ordered before treatment. T₄ replaces an older test known as the PBI (*protein-bound iodine*) test.

TEST TYPE: venous blood, capillary blood (from infant), chemistry

TEST OF: thyroid gland

TEST FOR: level in blood

HOW OFTEN: at birth; healthy women over 35 should be evaluated regularly.

NORMAL: **T₄** 2.8 - 13.5mcg/dl
    age 1-3 days  10.1 - 20.9 mcg/dl
        7-14       9.8 - 16.6 mcg/dl
       15-28     8.2 - 16.6 mcg/dl
      30-120   7.1 - 15 mcg/dl
**FT₄** 0.91 - 3 ng/dl
**PBI** 3.5 - 8.5 mcg/dl

> **TBG** 10 - 52 mcg/dl or
> 1.3 - 2 mg/dl by RIA.
> *Consult ranges given by your* lab.

HIGH:  $T_4$: overactive thyroid
TBG: liver disease

FALSE HIGH:

- <u>drugs</u>: birth control pills
- <u>environment</u>: cold weather, high altitude, pregnancy

LOW:  $T_4$: excess sex hormones (androgens and estrogens), underactive thyroid
TBG: chronic liver disease, kidney disease, overactive pituitary

FALSE LOW:

- <u>drugs</u>: epilepsy medication, steroids
- <u>environment</u>: aging, hot weather

COMMENTS: There is a third hormone produced by the thyroid gland -- *calcitonin*. Its role is not fully understood beyond the fact that it affects the two other thyroid hormones and lowers calcium levels in the blood. It may be tested for if thyroid cancer is suspected. Normal levels are below 0.155 ng/ml in men, 0.105 ng/ml in women.

*FTI (free thyroxine index)* measures the total level of thyroid hormones in the blood "by calculation," multiplying the level of $T_4$ times the level of $T_3$ uptake. This product, FTI ($T_7$), should be within 1.25 - 4.20 units. (Also known as *thyroid-hormone bonding ratio*.)

If you have had iodine given to you prior to the test, your doctor may measure your *basal metabolic rate* (BMR) instead of ordering the above tests. It is an indirect measure of thyroid function: the BMR measures the consumption of oxygen which indicates whether the thyroid is functioning normally.

### testosterone

DESCRIPTION: Secreted by the adrenal glands and testes (in men) or ovaries (in women), testosterone is an *androgen* hormone, primarily responsible for the development of "masculine" characteristics. If your lab sheet does not specify "free" from "total" levels, you can assume the value given is for the total level of testosterone.

Five blood samples are taken from women, three from men. Levels are highest in the morning (or, depending on your type of schedule, early in your waking cycle) and drop by midafternoon (50% in males, 30% in females).

TEST TYPE:      venous blood, chemistry

TEST OF:        pituitary gland

TEST FOR:       level in blood

HOW OFTEN:      with symptoms of infertility

NORMAL:         *Total*
- 194 - 1,200 ng/dl in men
- 6 - 95 ng/dl in women
- children before puberty:
    below 100 ng/dl in boys
    below 40 ng/dl in girls

*Free** (see COMMENTS, next page)

| Age | 20-29 | 30-39 | 40-49 | 50-59 | over 60 |
|---|---|---|---|---|---|
| male | 19-41 | 18-39 | 16-33 | 13-31 | 9-26 pg/ml |
| female | 0.9-3.2 | 0.8-3 | 0.6-2.5 | 0.3-2.7 | 0.2-2.2 |

*Free & Weakly Bound*\*
- 84 - 402 pg/ml in men
- 3 - 29 pg/ml in women
  *Consult ranges given by your lab..*

HIGH:          early sexual development, testicular tumor, adrenal disease/tumor, overactive thyroid, ovarian disease

LOW:           delayed sexual development, cancer (testes, prostate), liver disease, pituitary disease, testicular disease

FALSE LOW:
- <u>drugs</u>: estrogen therapy
- <u>medical</u>: surgical removal of testes

COMMENTS:  *Used to assess the biologically active testosterone in serum. Low levels are seen in women on birth control pills; high levels are seen in women with pronounced masculine characteristics (e.g., facial hair).

**thallium**
See **poisoning**, page 156.

## thyroid profile
### (thyroid function tests)

See individual tests:

- $T_3$ (triiodothyronine)
- $T_4$ (thyroxine)

DESCRIPTION: The thyroid is a gland which is part of the *endocrine system*. It secretes hormones ($T_3$ and $T_4$) which regulate metabolism, primarily in the breakdown of proteins, carbohydrates and fats. Such activity releases energy and, therefore, raises the temperature of the body.

However the manufacture of thyroid hormones requires dietary intake of iodine of 1 mg/week (from seafood, vegetables, eggs, dairy products, meat, iodized salt). It is from the iodine (which enters the blood at the small intestine and travels to thryoid gland where it accumulates) that thyroxine and triiodothyronine are made.

TEST TYPE: venous blood, chemistry

TEST OF: thyroid gland, metabolism

TEST FOR: level of thyroid hormones in blood

HOW OFTEN: at birth; with symptoms; healthy women over 35 should be evaluated more regularly

COMMENTS: For some labs, the *thyroid panel* will consist of $T_3$ **uptake** (page 179), $T_4$ **total** (page 181), and **free $T_4$ index** ($T_7$) by calculation (page 182).

# TIBC

## (total iron-binding capacity)

OTHER NAMES: serum transferrin, siderophilin

DESCRIPTION: Iron is attached to a protein (*transferrin*) in the blood. But just a measurement of the iron level is not all your doctor wants to know. TIBC measures how much your body <u>could</u> handle and what percent is already bound (what the laboratory calls "saturation").

 We get iron from what we eat and from recycled red blood cells. It is taken to the liver, spleen and bone marrow where it is either used or stored. The test for **iron** is usually done at the same time.

TEST TYPE:    venous blood, chemistry, iron studies

TEST OF:    iron metabolism

TEST FOR:    level of transferrin and percent that is attached (or *bound*) by iron

HOW OFTEN:    with symptoms

NORMAL:    188 - 450 mcg/dl
12 - 57% saturation (about 65 - 210 mcg/dl).
*Consult range given by your lab.*

HIGH:    anemia (due to iron deficiency), chronic blood loss

## TIBC (cont.)

**FALSE HIGH:**

- <u>diet</u>: iron deficiency
- <u>drugs</u>: birth control pills
- <u>environment</u>: pregnancy
- <u>medical</u>: recent blood transfusion

**LOW:** anemia, cancer, infection/infectious disease, iron overload (too much iron deposited into body tissue), kidney disease, liver disease

## TORCH

(**TO**xoplasmosis
**R**ubella
**C**ytomegalovirus
**H**erpes I & II tests)

**DESCRIPTION:** A group of tests run on a pregnant woman (or a newborn) to determine the child's immunity to these particular diseases. A pregnant woman with the proper antibodies will pass these to the fetus. Not all laboratories perform this series; not all doctors feel the tests are necessary.

**TEST TYPE:** venous blood, serology

**TEST OF:** immunity

**TEST FOR:** presence of antibodies

**HOW OFTEN:** during pregnancy (for the mother) or soon after birth (for the child)

**NORMAL:** positive in each of the 5 tests

ABNORMAL: negative (indicating a lack of immunity to the disease)

COMMENTS: All are **antibody** tests. In the past, many of the results have been inaccurate due to laboratory error. If your doctor orders the test, you might ask the lab if the kit they use is CDC (Centers for Disease Control & Prevention) tested and approved.

Your lab sheet might further specify the type of TORCH: whether IgG or IgM (e.g., "TORCH IgG panel"). Both are antibodies associated with the diseases: IgM will most likely be present if exposure is recent, IgG takes longer for antibodies to develop.

**total bili**
See **bilirubin** test, page 34.

**total protein**
See **protein**, page 162.

**transferrin**
See **TIBC**, page 186.

## triglycerides

DESCRIPTION: Fatty substance (lipid) used to store energy. In fact about 95% of fatty tissue is triglycerides. Like cholesterol, they can only be carried through the blood attached to a protein (as a *lipoprotein*). Even though triglycerides break down into fatty acids, the level of triglycerides is not a good predictor of coronary heart disease. It will, however, help to diagnose conditions that can be risk factors (see *VLDLs* in the **lipid panel**).

TEST TYPE:          venous blood, chemistry, lipid panel

TEST OF:            metabolism

TEST FOR:           level in blood

HOW OFTEN:          every 5 years

NORMAL:             10 - 200 mg/dl or
                    10 - 140 mg/dl for ages 0-29
                    10 - 150 mg/dl for ages 30-39
                    10 - 160 mg/dl for ages 40-49
                    10 - 190 mg/dl for ages 50-59
                    *Consult ranges given by your lab.*

HIGH:               primarily a disorder of fat metabolism brought about by: alcoholism, autoimmune disease, diabetes, kidney disease, liver disease, pancreatic inflammation/disease, thyroid underactivity

FALSE HIGH:

- <u>drugs</u>: Since it is not known which drugs will affect the test, try to eliminate as many drugs as possible in the 24-hour period preceding the test.

- environment: ingestion of alcohol/food prior to test, pregnancy

LOW:           malnutrition, inability to metabolize lipoproteins properly

COMMENTS:    When **cholesterol** levels are normal, a high triglyceride level does *not* seem to increase the risk of heart attack. However, *Prevention* magazine (March, 1989) recommends that if your triglycerides are over 150, be sure your **HDL** (page 89) is over 40. This should give you sufficient protection from increasing the risk of heart attack.


**triple test**
See either **AFP** (page 9), unconjugated **estriol** (page 67), or **hCG** (page 86) tests, performed as an initial screen of fetal health.

## tumor markers

See individual tests:

*Enzymes*
- **acid phos**, page 5
- **alk phos**, page 19
- **LD**, page 110
- **PSA**, page 163

*Hormones*
- **hCG**, page 86

*Plasma Protein*
- **AFP**, page 9

Measures the presence of substances produced and secreted by tumor cells that are found in the blood of patients with specific types of tumors.

**urea n** (urea nitrogen)
See **BUN**, page 39.

## uric acid

### (serum uric acid)

DESCRIPTION: Waste by-product of cell breakdown, *uric acid* is a component of urine and appears in the bloodstream before being excreted.

TEST TYPE:      venous blood, chemistry

TEST OF:        kidney, metabolism

TEST FOR:       level in blood

HOW OFTEN:   regular physical exam

NORMAL:
- 4.0 - 8.5 mg/dl in men
- 2.3 - 7.3 mg/dl in women. *Consult range given by your lab.*

HIGH:   anemia, arthritis, red blood cell overproduction, high blood pressure, cancer, enzyme deficiency, gout, heart failure, infections, kidney damage, leukemia, liver disease, pneumonia, skin disease, toxemia from pregnancy, tumors

FALSE HIGH:
- <u>drugs</u>: alcohol, aspirin, blood pressure medication, chemotherapy, diuretics, gout medication, L-dopa (medication for Parkinson's disease), vitamin C
- <u>environment</u>: fever, radiation

LOW:   kidney disease, liver atrophy

FALSE LOW:   <u>drugs</u>: gout medication

## vitamin A

OTHER NAMES: *retinol*

DESCRIPTION: An essential nutrient taken from the food we eat (leafy green vegetables, yellow fruits/vegetables, eggs, poultry, meat, fish). It is derived from *carotene*, which can also be measured by a blood test. Important for reproduction, bone growth, vision (especially night vision), and formation of *epithelia* (the protective coatings around organs)

TEST TYPE:     venous blood

TEST OF:       carbohydrate metabolism

TEST FOR:      level in blood

HOW OFTEN:     with symptoms of metabolic imbalance

NORMAL:
- 30 - 95 mcg/dl for adults
- 30 - 80 mcg/dl for children

*carotene*:
- 50 - 200 mg/dl for adults
- 40 - 130 mg/dl for children
- 0 - 40 mg/dl for infants

HIGH:          diabetes, supplement overdose (of either vitamin A or carotene, see page 156)

LOW:           impaired fat absorption (hepatitis, kidney inflammation, malnutrition, pregnancy which suppresses carotene), dietary deficiency

## vitamin B

DESCRIPTION: An essential nutrient not produced by the body and which must be ingested daily.

TEST TYPE:     venous blood

TEST OF:     carbohydrate metabolism

TEST FOR:     level in blood

HOW OFTEN:     with symptoms of metabolic imbalance

**vitamin $B_1$:** thiamin(e), thiamine pyrophosphate, transketolase; largest amounts are found in yeast, meats, eggs, whole grains, beans.

NORMAL:     0.60 – 1.06 IU/gram of hemoglobin or
             1.5 – 4 mcg/100ml

HIGH:     Since you cannot overdose on water-soluble vitamins, high values mean only that your diet includes thiamine-rich foods. An abundance does not seem to interfere with normal metabolism and will be excreted in the urine.

LOW:     alcoholism, beriberi, cancer, pregnancy, overactive thyroid

FALSE LOW:

- <u>diet</u>: excessive intake of egg whites
- <u>drugs</u>: alcohol, antibiotics
- <u>environment</u>: vomiting, diarrhea, lactation (in nursing mothers)

**vitamin B₂:** riboflavin; in dairy products, liver, kidneys, fish, green leafy vegetables, legumes; important for growth and tissue function.

NORMAL:　　　　1.4 - 5 mcg/dl

LOW:　　　　　　1.2-1.4, known as "low riboflavin nutritional status": dietary deficiency, poor absorption of nutrients, stress

**vitamin B₆:** 3 compounds: pyridoxine, pyridoxal and pyridoxamine (active form is PLP, *pyridoxal phospate* -- lab sheet may just refer to "pyridoxal-5-phosphate"); essential for protein metabolism, cell growth, blood formation.

NORMAL:　　　　5 - 24 ng/ml

**vitamin B₁₂:** cyanocobalamin, cobalamin, antipernicious anemia factor, extrinsic factor

DESCRIPTION:　A water-soluble vitamin containing cobalt; it is not produced in the body but is essential for the body's health. It influences red cell production, body growth and the formation of genes. Derived from non-plant foods (meat, shellfish, milk products, eggs), so lacto-ovo-vegetarians need supplements. In addition to measuring blood levels, a *vitamin B₁₂ unsaturated binding capacity* test is available

　Usually evaluated along with the test for **folic acid**, page 74. You will not get accurate results if you do not fast before the test (for 10-12 hours) or if you have been given *radionuclides* (if you have had "nuclear scanning" tests).

NORMAL:　　　**blood level**
　　　　　　　　200 - 1,100 pg/ml or

150 - 810 pmol/l
*Indeterminate*
160 - 200 pg/ml
**binding capacity**
1000 - 2000 pg/ml
*Consult the ranges given by your lab.*

HIGH: blood disease, congestive heart failure, diabetes, chronic kidney failure (hepatitis), leukemia, liver disease (cirrhosis), obesity

FALSE HIGH: <u>diet</u>: too much $B_{12}$ in diet or by supplements

LOW: anemia, central nervous system damage, dietary deficiency, intestinal malabsorption*, overactive thyroid

FALSE LOW:

- <u>drugs</u>: barbiturates, birth control pills, chemotherapy drugs (methotrexate), diuretics (triamterene), epilepsy medication (phenytoin), malaria drugs (pyrimethamine, trimethoprim), TB medication (aminosalicylic acid, cycloserine)
- <u>environment</u>: pregnancy, surgical removal of stomach, agitation of sample

COMMENTS: *When we eat $B_{12}$ (called the *extrinsic factor* because it comes from outside the body), it combines in the stomach with a specialized protein called an *intrinsic factor* (because it is made inside the body in the gastric glands). This complex travels through the intestine to absorption sites where $B_{12}$ separates from the intrinsic factor and enters the bloodstream for delivery to body tissues. Some $B_{12}$ is stored in the liver; any excess is excreted.

## vitamin C

OTHER NAMES: ascorbic acid

DESCRIPTION: A water-soluble vitamin found in citrus fruits, berries, tomatoes, raw cabbage, green peppers, green leafy vegetables. It is needed to maintain healthy cartilage and bone as well as for iron absorption, folic acid metabolism, healing from injury/infection.

TEST TYPE:         venous blood

TEST OF:           carbohydrate metabolism

TEST FOR:          level in blood

HOW OFTEN:         with symptoms of metabolic imbalance

NORMAL:            0.2-2.0 mg/dl

HIGH:              although non-toxic in high doses, can lead to diarrhea or vomiting, gout, iron toxicity, kidney stones, medication interference, urinary problems (see page 157)

LOW:               anemia, blood vessel fragility, fever, infection, joint abnormalities, pregnancy, scurvy

## vitamin D

DESCRIPTION: A fat-soluble vitamin produced in the skin from the sun's UV rays as well as occurring in food (fish liver oils, egg yolks, liver, butter); important for bone growth by regulating **calcium** and **phosphorus**.

TEST TYPE:       venous blood

TEST OF:         carbohydrate metabolism

TEST FOR:        level in blood

HOW OFTEN:       with symptoms of metabolic imbalance

**Vitamin D3**: cholecalciferol

NORMAL:

- 10 - 80 ng/ml *25-hydroxycholecalciferol* (the substance vitamin D3 converts to in the blood) in summer
- 10 - 42 ng/ml in winter

HIGH:            supplement overdose (page 157), sensitivity to vitamin D

**Vitamin D(1,25 dihydroxy):** 25-hydroxy-vitamin D, serum 25-OH-D (biologically active form of vitamin D)

NORMAL:          10 - 55 ng/ml adults
                 17 - 54 ng/ml ages 1 to 18
                 8 - 21 ng/ml below age 1

LOW:             poor diet, too little sun, rickets (softening of the bones), malabsorption (from liver/pancreas disease, celiac disease, cystic fibrosis, stomach/bowel removal, drug interaction from hormones or sedatives)

## vitamin E

OTHER NAMES: alpha-tocopherol

DESCRIPTION: A fat-soluble vitamin which means it accumulates in the body and can become toxic (see page 157). As a vitamin it must be ingested, preferably in the food we eat (vegetable oils, nuts, wheat germ, leafy green vegetables) or from supplements. It protects the body's tissues from the effects of *free radicals* (page 129) which is why it is called an *antioxidant* (it helps to preserve cell membranes from oxidation, the normal action of oxygen).

TEST TYPE: venous blood

TEST OF: carbohydrate metabolism

TEST FOR: level in blood

HOW OFTEN: with symptoms of metabolic imbalance

NORMAL: 5 - 20 mcg/ml

HIGH: overdose (probably from supplements, see page 157)

LOW: anemia, malabsorption of fats; (symptoms of deficiency include unsteadiness and color changes in the eye)

## vitamin K

DESCRIPTION: A fat-soluble vitamin needed by the body for proper blood clotting (vitamin K is broken down in the colon then sent to the liver to make *blood clotting factors*). Present in the leaves of plants so all leafy vegetables will be a dietary source. Sometimes newborns don't have enough of the intestinal bacteria needed to process vitamin K.

TEST TYPE: venous blood

TEST OF: carbohydrate metabolism

TEST FOR: level in blood

HOW OFTEN: with symptoms of metabolic imbalance

NORMAL: 0.09 - 2.2 ng/ml

HIGH: overdose (probably from supplements, see page 157)

LOW: bile disorders (e.g., obstruction), internal bleeding, malabsorption

FALSE LOW: <u>drugs</u>: antibiotics (which kill the necessary bacteria in the colon)

# WBC

## (white blood cell count)

OTHER NAMES: leukocyte (or leucocyte) count

DESCRIPTION: Cells designed to attack infection or any invasive, foreign substance. The actual count will vary throughout the day: lowest in the early morning (when you have been still for awhile), highest in the afternoon (after you have been active for awhile)

TEST TYPE:     venous blood, hematology, CBC

TEST OF:       blood, immune system

TEST FOR:      number and appearance of cells

HOW OFTEN:     regular physical exam

NORMAL:

- 3,500 - 11,000 $mm^3$ in adults
- higher from infancy to 2 year old. *Consult ranges given by your lab.*

HIGH:          bacterial infection, blood disorders, leukemia, tissue damage

FALSE HIGH:

- <u>drugs</u>: anesthesia, antibiotics, arthritis medication, aspirin, gout medication, malaria medication
- <u>environment</u>: childbirth, emotional distress, menstruation, muscular exercise, pregnancy, trauma

LOW:                alcoholism, anemia, blood toxicity, bone marrow
                    failure, diabetes, viral infection

FALSE LOW:

- <u>drugs</u>: antibiotics, antiinflammatory medication,
  chemotherapy drugs, sedative, thyroid medication
- <u>environment</u>: dietary deficiencies

COMMENTS: The WBC count can vary by 2,000 mm$^3$ from the indirect environmental factors of digestion, exercise, infection, smoking, and stress.

## WBC diff

### (white blood cell differential count)

DESCRIPTION: There are 3 classes of white blood cells (WBCs): *granulocytes, monocytes* and *lymphocytes.*
   Lab sheets may further distinguish the cells into the six types listed below. For the test, these cells are isolated and measured. Each cell type may show two values: *%* and *absolute.* The *percentage* number is relative to the total WBC sample: the percentage of the total that are "basophils," for example. *Absolute* value refers to the actual cell count in numbers.

TEST TYPE:     capillary blood, hematology, CBC

TEST OF:       immune system

TEST FOR:      amount, proportionately, of each cell type

HOW OFTEN:     suspected blood infection or toxicity

**WBC diff** (cont.)

| NORMAL: | % | absolute |
|---|---|---|
| bands | 0 - 3 | 0 - 330 mm$^3$ |
| basophils | trace - 2 | 1 - 220 mm$^3$ |
| eosinophils | 0.3 - 7 | 10 - 770 mm$^3$ |
| lymphocytes | 16 - 43 | 560 - 4,370 mm$^3$ |
| monocytes | trace - 10 | 1 - 1,100 mm$^3$ |
| neutrophils | 47 - 77 | 1,645 - 8,470 mm$^3$ |

*Consult ranges given by your lab.*

Imbalances are referred to as "*shifts*" to the left or right, depending on which cell type increases.

Newborns start off with adult proportions but lymphocytes very quickly increase and neutrophils will decrease. From ages 6 to 17, values will vary by gender: girls having slightly more neutrophils and basophils than boys, and slightly fewer lymphocytes, monocytes, and eosinophils. Adult proportions reappear after adolescence.

## GRANULOCYTES

OTHER NAMES: polymorphonucleocytes, PMN, polys

*Granulocytes* are the first line of defense against disease. They are the first to arrive at the site of injury or infection and are called "phago-cytic" because they eat or otherwise destroy unrecognized matter. They are made in the bone marrow. The darkest cells on the front cover are granulocytes (notice the dark granules contained within the cells). Four of the six types of white blood cells usually tested for are granulocytes: **bands, neutrophils, eosinophils** and **basophils**.

## • bands

OTHER NAMES: stabs (because of having a distinctive curved nucleus)

DESCRIPTION: an immature neutrophil

HIGH: bacterial infection

COMMENTS: Because it takes about a week for neutrophils to mature (and then they only live a few hours), supplies are kept on hand in the form of *bands*. They are stored in the bone marrow (where blood cells are made); the number given in the **WBC** differential test is but a fraction of what is available.

In a bacterial infection, neutrophils and bands are both increased, producing a "shift to the left" in the differential.

## • neutrophils
**(neutral-staining multinucleated cells)**

Because neutrophils eat bacteria (among other microorganisms), if you are prone to bacterial infections, your doctor may order specialized tests to see how effective your neutrophils are.

HIGH: local tissue death (from burns, cancer, heart attack), infection, inflammation and inflammatory disease

FALSE HIGH: environment: burns, stress (from surgery, exercise, pregnancy, childbirth, emotional crisis)

## WBC diff, Granulocytes (cont.)

LOW:  infection, lupus; low levels can also make people more susceptible to bacterial infection

FALSE LOW:

- <u>environment</u>: radiation
- <u>nutrition</u>: vitamin $B_{12}$ or folic acid deficiency

- **eosinophils**
**(acid-staining multinucleated cells)**

OTHER NAMES: eos, acidophils

HIGH:  adrenal insufficiency, allergies, autoimmune disease, cancer, leukemia, parasites, skin disease

LOW:  Cushing's disease

FALSE LOW:  <u>environment</u>: stress

COMMENTS: Eosinophils eat parasites as well as moderating the effects of inflammation.

- **basophils**
**(basic-staining multinucleated cells)**

HIGH:  blood poisoning, cancer, leukemia, underactive thyroid

FALSE HIGH:  chronic hypersensitivity (for example, allergies)

LOW:              overactive thyroid

FALSE LOW:     <u>environment</u>: pregnancy, ovulation, stress

COMMENTS:  Basophils are huge and do their work in our "barrier tissues" (skin and mucous membranes).  They make the histamine that causes the congestion when we have a cold.

# MONOCYTES

*Monocytes* follow granulocytes to the site of injury (and stay around where there is chronic infection).  They are made in the bone marrow and circulate in the blood as monocytes.  When they get to the infected tissue, they develop into *macrophages.*

OTHER NAMES: monos, macrophages, tissue phagocytes

DESCRIPTION:  Large white blood cells that eat foreign substances, remember what they eat, and pass this information along to lymphocytes. (Granulocytes simply vaporize the substance.)

HIGH:             blood vessel disease, cancer, infection (fungal, viral), leukemia, tuberculosis

COMMENTS:  Macrophages have an important function in addition to their scavenging.  They also deliver proteins to tissue throughout the body.

## LYMPHOCYTES

*Lymphocytes* are the management part of the immune system: they remember what invaded the body before, they direct production of antibodies and determine when health has been restored. In other words, they are what give us immunity to a particular disease. They include **B lymphocytes**, **T lymphocytes**, and **NK cells**.

- **B lymphocytes**

OTHER NAMES: bone marrow-derived lymphocytes, B cells, humoral immune system

DESCRIPTION: They are made in the bone marrow but mature in the lymph glands. These are the cells that produce antibodies which neutralize specific disease-causing organisms. They are directed (turned on and off) by T cells. B cells circulate in the blood and create antibodies (gamma globulins, **immunoglobulins**, Igs), that class of protein which assists the immune system in fighting infection. See **globulin** test, page 80. Gamma globulins can be further isolated into IgG ("immunoglobulin G"), IgA, IgM, IgE and IgD.

NORMAL: 10% - 20% of total white blood cell count. *Consult range given by your lab.*

HIGH: anemia, leukemia, tumors

LOW: immunoglobulin deficiency diseases (e.g., AIDS), leukemia

## • T lymphocytes

OTHER NAMES: thymus-derived lymphocytes, T cells, cellular
immune system

DESCRIPTION: They are made in the bone marrow but mature in
the thymus gland. There are 2 types: T4 (T-helper cells, CD4 cells)
signal the B cells to produce antibodies; T8 (T-suppressor cells) stop
production when no more antibodies are needed. T4 cells are what
hold the memory of previous foreign bodies and call out defenses with
any new encounter of these bodies.

TEST OF: blood, thymus gland

HOW OFTEN: When HIV is present, your doctor will begin
monitoring the level of T4 cells and the ratio of T4
to T8 cells.

NORMAL: 68% - 75% of total white blood cell count.
*Consult range given by your lab.*

700 - 1,300 ml (T4 cells)
**T4/T8 ratio**: 2/1. There should be, roughly, twice
the number of T4 cells as T8 cells.

HIGH: immune disease, infection (bacterial, viral),
leukemia, measles, tumors

LOW: AIDS, suppression of immune response (from a
wide variety of diseases which suppress the T-
cells), leukemia

**T lymphocytes** (cont.)

FALSE LOW:

- <u>drugs</u>: steroids
- <u>environment</u>: prolonged illness

- **natural killer cells**
**(NK cells)**

DESCRIPTION: They may be a type of lymphocyte. They are directed, however, by T cells and are part of the cellular immune system (because they directly attack cells instead of producing antibodies to attack). Specifically, they attack some tumor cells and some virus-infected cells.

### Western blot

DESCRIPTION: A type of test in which an electric current is run though the sample and the pattern of migration is interpreted (known as *electrophoresis*). This is the second test for HIV, confirming a positive **ELISA**.

TEST TYPE:     venous blood, serology

TEST OF:     blood

HOW OFTEN:     with a positive ELISA test (page 64) or exposure to an infectious agent

NORMAL:     negative

FALSE NEGATIVE: too early to detect antibodies

POSITIVE:        presence of or exposure to pathogen is highly likely
<ins>indeterminate</ins>: laboratory cannot tell, test should
be repeated in 3 months

FALSE POSITIVE: laboratory error (including switched samples)

COMMENTS: The *Western* in the name comes about as follows. The "inventor" of this *type* of test was Dr. E.M. Southern and the test was named the "Southern blot." Another inventor reversed Southern's method (for a different test) and paid tribute to Southern by naming the new test the "Northern blot." The "Western blot" name continues this tribute as the test is similar to Southern's. (From Pinckney, see *Bibliography*.)

## zinc

DESCRIPTION: A metallic element and essential nutrient which comes from our diet (water, meat, seafood, dairy products, whole grains, nuts, legumes). Most (75%-88%) of the zinc in the bloodstream is in the red blood cells and the levels rise and fall at regular intervals during the day (peak values seem to be at 9 am and 6 pm).

TEST TYPE: venous blood, chemistry

TEST OF: blood

TEST FOR: level in blood

HOW OFTEN: with symptoms

NORMAL: 60 - 150 mcg/dl

HIGH: supplement overdose, environmental exposure (see page 157)

LOW: anemia, heart attack, kidney failure, liver disease, rheumatoid arthritis, drug interference (e.g., corticosteroids); retards growth and sexual development, enlargement of the spleen. You can get a deficiency from diets rich in cereals (phytates) that bind zinc.

# GLOSSARY

**acid** Any substance in the body's fluids with a pH below 7. It reacts with a "base" (an alkaline substance) to maintain the proper acid-base balance of the fluids.

**Addison's disease** "Wasting" (weakness, weight loss) due to underactivity of the adrenal gland.

**alkali** A chemical substance in the body's fluids with a pH above 7. It reacts with an "acid" to maintain the proper acid-base balance of the fluids.

**amino acid** An organic compound which links with other amino acids to form a protein molecule. Proteins are defined by the order of their constituent amino acids.

**amniocentesis** A test performed on pregnant women to diagnose Down syndrome in the fetus. Cells from the amniotic fluid (in the placenta) are drawn out with a needle, thus creating the risk of miscarriage.

**analgesic** A pain medication.

**androgen** A hormone that produces some masculine characteristics.

**anemia** When too little oxygen is carried in the blood, there won't be enough to go around. This results in the body slowing down to conserve what oxygen there is (so you will feel tired and "run down").

**anesthetic** A drug used to dull feeling in a particular area (*local anesthesia*) or to cause a loss of consciousness (*general anesthesia*).

**aneurysm** A deformation of a part of a blood vessel. The wall may be thin and unable to keep its shape; the pressure of the blood will push out the wall (which will either break or cause obstruction).

**antacid** Anti-acid, literally "against acid." A compound that neutralizes acid in the stomach. Hence, aspirin is sometimes coated with antacids to "buffer" the effect of the aspirin.

**antibacterial** A drug that kills bacteria. Its function is exactly that of an antibiotic, but it kills bacteria in a slightly different way.

**antibiotic** A drug that kills bacteria in the body.

**antibody** A protein substance made by white blood cells to get rid of unfamiliar substances (*antigens*) in the blood. The body assumes anything unfamiliar will cause illness. In most cases, once antibodies are made the threat of illness disappears. The purpose of vaccinating children is to give them specific antibodies without waiting for them to make antibodies "naturally" (when the illness is introduced into their blood).

**anticholinergic** Medication that increases blood pressure, constricts blood vessels or slows the secretion of digestive fluids by blocking the passage of nerve impulses through the parasympathetic nerves.

**antigen** A foreign (unfamiliar) substance in the blood which provokes white blood cells into making antibodies.

**antihistamine** Medication that blocks the production of *histamine* (which dilates blood vessels).

**antiseptic** A chemical substance that kills germs (bacteria, fungi, viruses). So, for example, an antibiotic is an antiseptic.

**ARC (AIDS-related complex)** An illness ultimately caused by HIV infection. Can precede AIDS, although not always.

**ARC-defining diagnosis** One or more infections (thrush, *oral hairy leukoplakia*, shingles, ITP -- *idiopathic thrombocytopenic purpura*) AND/OR the presence of HIV antibodies in your blood AND a low number of T4 white blood cells. Persistent ill health (fatigue, weight loss, fever, diarrhea) may be used to diagnose ARC when HIV is present.

**arterial blood**  Blood taken from an artery (usually from the wrist). Arterial blood contains oxygen on its way to body cells.

**asthma**  Difficulty breathing because the air passages have spasmed or the membranes are swollen.  Usually a chronic condition which can be brought on by allergies.

**autonomic nervous system**  Regulates involuntary action; consists of *sympathetic* and *parasympathetic* nervous systems.

**bacteria**  A variety of small organisms which can live in our body normally (to aid digestion, for example) or invade the body (to cause disease or infection).

**basal metabolism**  The minimum amount of energy used by the body. There is a fairly old test which measures this.

**bilirubin**  The pigment (color) formed during digestion which is excreted along with the waste products from digestion (including discarded red blood cells which are brown like dried blood and are what makes a stool brown).

**blood**  The fluid that circulates throughout the body, consisting of red and white cells floating in a liquid (plasma).

**blood type**  Type A, type B, type AB or type O, according to what proteins (*antigens*) are on the surface of the red blood cell.

**BSP (Bromsulphalein test)**  A dye injected into the body and used to monitor liver function.

**BUN (blood urea nitrogen)**  See test, page 39.

**capillary**  A microscopic blood vessel with very thin walls through which oxygen is passed to the body's tissues.

**capillary blood**  Blood taken from a capillary at the periphery (outer edges) of the body, usually gotten with a prick to a fingertip (see "fingerstick").

**catalyst**  A substance which helps a chemical reaction to take place but is not itself absorbed in the reaction.  Enzymes, for example, are catalysts in the digestion of food.

**CBC (complete blood count)** See test, page 47.

**cellular immune system** The lymphocytes, those white blood cells which defend the body against disease by attacking disease cells directly.

**central nervous system** Brain and spinal cord.

**chemotherapy** Drug therapy; treating disease with chemical substances (drugs).

**complement system** Part of our immune defense, *complements* are proteins that circulate in the blood in an inactive state looking for intruders. Once activated, they prepare the way for the rest of the immune system to work.

**Crohn's disease** Chronic inflammation of the bowel.

**Cushing's disease (Cushing's syndrome)** Obesity and muscular weakness.

**decongestant** A substance that relieves a stuffy nose, usually by constricting the blood vessels.

**dehydration** Excessive loss of water from the body; particularly threatening to children with severe diarrhea.

**depressant** A drug that slows down the central nervous system.

**diabetes** A metabolic disorder in which the body cannot break down and absorb sugar normally.

**Down syndrome** A genetic disorder manifested by varying degrees of mental retardation.

**electrolyte** A particle that conducts electricity (so the particle will have either a positive or negative charge).

**electrophoresis** A type of test in which an electric current is passed through the blood sample and the resulting pattern of migration used for diagnosis.

**emetic** Medication that is meant to cause vomiting.

**enzyme** Protein made by the body that helps a particular chemical reaction take place. (Chemical reactions break down food and other substances into simpler forms that can be absorbed by the body.) Enzymes are normally found in cells and tissues.

**estrogens**  The hormones that help produce female characteristics.

**fingerstick**  A drop or two of blood taken by making a small puncture in the tip of a finger.  If some other part of the body is used, the heel, for example, of a newborn, the puncture will be called a "heelstick."

**Gaucher's disease**  A genetic disorder characterized by spleen and liver enlargement and abnormal bone growth.

**glaucoma**  An eye disease in which too much fluid presses on the eyeball.

**Grave's disease**  A disorder of the thyroid gland in which too much of the thyroid hormone is produced making the thyroid overactive.

**hemorrhage**  Excessive bleeding.

**HIV**  Human immunodeficiency virus. See page 95.

**Hodgkin's disease**  A type of cancer which starts in the lymph nodes and may progress into the liver and lungs.

**hormone**  A chemical substance made in one of the endocrine glands (adrenal, parathyroid, pituitary, thyroid).

**humoral immune system**  Part of the immune defense system. Consists of antibodies circulating in the bloodstream.

**hypervolemia**  Too much blood is circulating through the body.

**hypnotic**  A drug that induces sleep; stronger than a sedative.

**hypovolemia**  Too little blood is circulating through the body.

**IFA (indirect fluorescent-antibody assay)**  A type of antibody test in which a fluorescent compound attaches to a designated antibody, thus allowing a blood sample to be easily analyzed.

**immune defensive system**  How the body protects itself from disease.  Consists of the "humoral immune system" (antibodies, etc. circulating in the bloodstream) and the "cellular immune system" (the lymphocytes) working together.

**immunoglobulin** Antibody.

**infection** The growth of a (possibly toxic) foreign substance in the body and the reaction of the immune system.

**intravenous** "Within the vein," literally. Often referred to as an "IV," a solution is given *intravenously* when it is administered continuously into the vein with a needle.

**intrinsic factor** A protein in the stomach that binds with vitamin $B_{12}$ to allow absorption through the intestine.

**lupus** *Systemic lupus erythematosus*, SLE, is a chronic inflammatory connective tissue disease that affects the skin, joints, and muscles.

**lymphoma** Tumor of the lymph glands.

**macrophage** "Big eater" of foreign bodies. A white blood cell (monocyte type) that matures into a scavenger cell in the body's tissues.

**metabolism** The process by which food and oxygen are used by the body to provide energy.

**microphage** "Little eater" of foreign bodies. A white blood cell (granulocyte type) that scavenges.

**molecular diagnostics** A technique of examining the body's fluids (blood, urine, saliva, etc.) for genetic material: genes which have mutated (changed from normal into abnormal) and might then give rise to cancer cells, viral RNA which directly proves the presence of a specific virus. Identifying such genes will make early diagnosis of illness possible.

**natural killer (NK) cells** White blood cells that puncture some tumor and virus-infected cells, causing them to die.

**occult blood** This refers to bleeding that cannot easily be seen. When the term is used on your lab sheet, it means your urine, feces or some other bodily excretion has been examined for the presence of blood. (There should be none; the test value should be "negative.")

**opportunistic infection** Usually we think of infections as arising from a foreign substance, something outside the body that gets in and mobilizes the immune system. But many disease-causing substances can live in the body and are suppressed by the normal activities of the immune system. If the white blood cells which direct the immune system (the T lymphocytes) are damaged, then those formerly harmless substances can take over and do a lot of damage.

**oxalate** A cleansing agent made from *oxalic acid* and found in car radiator cleaners, laundry bleach, fabric manufacture/ cleaning; occurs naturally in some house plants (*dieffenbachia, philodendron*).

**Paget's disease** A type of cancer involving the ducts of the breast, sometimes accompanied by inflammation of the skin.

**parasympathetic nervous system** Opposes the action of the *sympathetic nervous system* by stimulating digestion, slowing the heart, dilating blood vessels.

**Parkinson's disease** Progressive deterioration of the central nervous system usually recognizable by the loss of motor function and onset of tremors, spasms and paralysis.

**pathogen** Any agent that causes disease.

**PCR (polymerase chain reaction)** Test used in molecular diagnostics to identify a particular virus from its genetic material in the blood.

**peripheral blood** Blood taken from a capillary (by a fingerstick, or heelstick on newborns).

**plasma** The liquid portion of *unclotted* blood which includes dissolved vitamins, minerals, gases, sugars, hormones, antibodies, fats, proteins, and traces of food and drugs.

**progesterone** Another hormone helping to produce female sexual characteristics.

**PSP (Phenolsulfonphthalein test)** A dye injected into the body and used to monitor liver function.

**pulmonary embolism** Blood clot which travels from the leg to the lung. Can be fatal when it blocks blood flow to the heart.

**radioimmunoassay** Direct measure of minute quantities of substances in the blood or urine, formerly not directly measurable.

**random specimen** Urine sample which is collected at any time.

**RIA** Radioimmunoassay.

**Reye's syndrome** Respiratory infection in children which can be fatal, particularly when aspirin is given.

**salt** The "neutralized" product of an acid reacting with an alkali (base).

**scavenger cells** White blood cells that eat or destroy foreign particles.

**serum** The liquid portion of *clotted* blood which, like plasma, includes dissolved vitamins, minerals, gases, sugars, hormones, antibodies, fats, proteins, and traces of food and drugs.

**sympathetic nervous system** Prepares our body for stress by increasing the heart rate, increasing blood flow to the muscles and decreasing blood flow to the skin.

**testosterone** A hormone helping to create male sexual characteristics.

**thrombin** A blood clotting substance made from thromboplastin, prothrombin and calcium.

**thrombophlebitis** An infected thrombosis.

**thrombosis** Excessive blood clotting.

**titration** An antibody test. A blood sample is progressively diluted and tested for its ability to neutralize a live virus introduced to the sample. The highest dilution which neutralizes the virus is called an *antibody titer*.

**vasoconstrictor** Any substance able to narrow (constrict) the blood vessels.

**vasodilator** Any substance able to enlarge (dilate) the blood vessels.

**venous blood** Blood taken from a vein (usually with a needle). Venous blood contains carbon dioxide on its way to the lungs to be exhaled.

## Alphabetical list of drugs mentioned in the text:

acetazolamide (glaucoma, epilepsy)
aminosalicylic acid (TB medication)
ammonium chloride (diuretic)
azathioprine (immunosuppressant)
bacille Calmette-Guerin vaccine (chemotherapy drugs)
cephalosporins (antibiotics)
chloral hydrate (hypnotic, sedative)
chloramphenicol (antibiotics)
chlorpromazine (tranquilizer)
chlorpropamide (diabetes medication)
clofibrate (antihyperlipidemic: lipid reducer)
corticosteroids (antiinflammatory, hormone replacement therapy,
      cancer drugs)
corticotropin (anticonvulsant, antiemetic)
cortisone (antiinflammatory)
cycloserine (TB medication)
dactinomycin (antibiotics)
dimercaperol (poisoning antidote)
ethacrynic acid (diuretic),
ethosuximide (anticonvulsant, epilepsy medication)
furazolidone (antibacterial, antiprotozoal)
furosemide (diuretic)
glutethimide (hypnotic, sedative)
griseofulvin (antibiotic, antifungal)
hydralazine (vasodilator, blood pressure reducer)
isoniazid (antibacterial, TB medication)
mephenytoin (anticonvulsant: epilepsy)
methicillin (antibacterial)
methotrexate (chemotherapy drugs)
methyldopa (blood pressure reducer)
methylprednisolone (hormones)
methysergide (vasoconstrictor)

oxyphenbutazone, (arthritis, gout)
para-aminosalicylic acid (TB antibiotic)
paraldehyde (hypnotic, sedative)
penicillin (antibiotic)
phenylbutazone (analgesic, antipyretic, antiinflammatory, gout
    medication, rheumatoid arthritis & other rheumatoid
    conditions)
phenylbutazone (rheumatoid conditions, arthritis, gout)
phenytoin (anticonvulsant: epilepsy medication; antiarrhythmic:
    cardiac depressant)
primidone (anticonvulsant, epilepsy medication)
procainamide (anesthetic)
propylthiouracil (thyroid inhibitor)
pyrimethamine (malaria drug)
quinidine (cardiac depressive, antimalarial)
reserpine (antihypertensive: blood pressure reducer, sedative)
salicylates (analgesic, antipyretic, antiinflammatory)
streptomycin (antibiotic)
sulfonamide (antibiotic, sulfa drugs)
tetracyclines (antibiotic)
thiazides (diuretic)
triamterene (diuretic)
trimethadione (anticonvulsant-analgesic: epilepsy medication)
trimethoprim (malaria drug)
vasopressin (ADH, antidiuretic hormone, diabetes medication, blood
    vessel constrictor)

## Alphabetical list of abbreviations used in the text:

# BIBLIOGRAPHY

Barnhart, Edward R., publisher *Physician's Desk Reference*, 44th edition (Oradel, NJ: Medical Economics Company, 1990).

Bartlett, John G., MD & Ann K. Kinkbeiner *The Guide to Living with HIV Infection* (Baltimore: The Johns Hopkins University Press, 1991).

Brunner, Lillian S. & Doris S. Suddarth *Lippincott Manual of Nursing Practice*, 2nd edition (Philadelphia: J.B. Lippincott Company, 1974).

Centers for Disease Control *1993 Revised Classification System for HIV Infection and Expanded Surveillance Case Definition for AIDS Among Adolescents and Adults* MMWR 1992:41, 1-23.

Centers for Disease Control *1994 Revised Classification System for Human Immunodeficiency Virus Infection in Children Less Than 13 Years of Age* MMWR 1994:43, 1-10.

*Clinical Laboratory Tests: Values and Implications* 2nd edition (Springhouse, PA: Springhouse Corporation, 1995).

Consumer Reports Books editors *Medicine Show* 5th edition (Mount Vernon, NY: Consumers Union, 1983).

*Dorland's Illustrated Medical Dictionary* 28th edition (Philadelphia: W.B. Saunders Company, 1994).

*Encyclopedia Britannica* 15th edition (Chicago: Encyclopedia Britannica, Inc., 1991).

*Everything You Need to Know About Medical Tests* (Springhouse, PA: Springhouse Corporation, 1996).

Flanders, Stephen A. & Carl N. *AIDS*, Library in a Book Series (New York: Facts On File, 1991).

Garb, Solomon, MD *Laboratory Tests in Common Use* 6th edition (New York: Springer Publishing Company, 1976).

Govoni, Laura E., PhD, RN & Janice E. Hayes, RhD, RN *Drugs and Nursing Implications* 2nd edition (New York: Apleton-Century-Crofts, 1971).

Greenspan, Debra *AIDS and the Mouth: Diagnosis and Management of Oral Lesions* (Munksgaard, 1990).

*Illustrated Guide to Diagnostic Tests* 2nd edition (Springhouse, PA: Springhouse Corporation, 1998).

Kusinitz, Marc *Poisons and Toxins* (New York: Chelsea House Publishers, 1993).

Lyon, Jeff & Peter Gorner *Altered Fates: Gene Therapy and the Retooling of Human Life* (New York: W.W. Norton & Co., 1995).

Mindell, Earl L., RPh, PhD *Earl Mindell's Pill Bible* (New York: Bantam Books, 1984).

Mayo Clinic, Reference Laboratory of the, *1986 Test Catalog* (Rochester, MN: Mayo Medical Laboratories, 1986).

*Merck Manual of Diagnosis and Therapy, The* 15th edition (Rahway, NJ: Merck & Company, 1987)

*Merck Manual of Medical Information, The* Home Edition (Whitehouse Station, NJ: Merck Research Laboratories, 1997).

Morris, William, editor *American Heritage Dictionary of the English Language* College Edition (Boston: Houghton Mifflin Company, 1979).

Nelson-Anderson, Danette L., RN, BSN & Cynthia V. Waters *Genetic Connections: A Guide to Documenting Your Individual and Family Health History* (Washington, MO: Sonters Publishing, 1995).

Nourse, Alan E., MD *AIDS* (New York: Franklin Watts, 1989)

Pagana, Kathleen D., RN, MSN & Timothy J. Pagana, MD *Understanding Medical Testing* (St. Louis: Times Mirror New American Library, 1983).

Pinckney, Cathey & Edward R. Pinckney, MD *Patient's Guide to Medical Tests* 3rd edition (New York: Facts On File, 1986).

Schoub, Barry D., MD, DSc *AIDS & HIV in Perspective: A Guide to Understanding the Virus and its Consequences* (Cambridge, UK: Cambridge University Press, 1994).

Silverman, Harold M., PharmD & Gilbert I. Simon, DSc *Pill Book* (New York: Bantam Books, 1979).

Sobel, David S. MD & Tom Ferguson, MD *People's Book of Medical Tests* (New York: Summit Books, 1985).

*Testing for HIV: What Your Lab Results Mean* (Lake Grove, NY: TBL, 1995).

Tortora, Gerard J. & Nicholas P. Anagnostakos *Principles of Anatomy and Physiology* 3$^{rd}$ edition (New York: Harper & Row, 1981).

Turkington, Carol *Poisons and Antidotes* (New York: Facts On File, 1994).

Tver, David F. & Percy Russell, PhD *The Nutrition and Health Encyclopedia* (New York: Van Nostrand Reinhold Company, 1981).

Vargo, Marc, MS *The HIV Test: What You Need to Know to Make an Informed Decision* (New York: Pocket Books, 1992).

Ward, Darrell E., MS *The AmFAR AIDS Handbook: The Complete Guide to Understanding HIV and AIDS* (New York: W.W. Norton & Company, 1999).

Winter, Ruth *A Consumer's Dictionary of Household, Yard and Office Chemicals* (New York: Crown Publishers, 1992).

Wittman, Karl S., PhD & John C. Thomas, BA *Medical Laboratory Skills* Nursing and Allied Health Series (New York: McGraw-Hill Book Company, 1977).

Wolfe, Sidney M., MD & Rose-Ellen Hope, RPh *Worst Pills Best Pills II: The Older Adult's Guide to Avoiding Drug-Induced Death or Illness* (Washington, DC: Public Citizen's Health Research Group, 1993).

# INDEX

To order directly from the publisher, include the following information with a check or money order and send to:

Technical Books for the Layperson, Inc.
P. O. Box 391
Lake Grove, NY 11755-0391

Name_____

Address _____

_____

City_____

State _____ Zip Code _____

Phone __(      )_____

*Common Blood Tests* $20
  Please send ____ copies.      _____
  Add $2.50 first book for S/H
     $.50 each additional book    _____

Subtotal                  _____

NY residents add 8.25% sales tax  _____

TOTAL ENCLOSED       _____

The books will be mailed "Book Rate" which takes, according to the Post Office, ten days to two weeks.